INDULGE YOURSELF WITH PAMPERING REGIMENS INSPIRED BY THOSE USED AT THE WORLD'S MOST LUXURIOUS SPAS . . .

CANYON RANCH SPA IN THE BERKSHIRES . . .
This highly respected spa harnesses the healing energy of the sea with *Digita laminaria,* or kelp, imported from the northwestern shores of France. You can share in the multiple benefits of a similar mineral-rich wrap that is especially wonderful for dry or damaged skin . . . right in your own tub.

GREEN VALLEY SPA, UTAH . . .
In southwest Utah's spectacular desert, this retreat, perched on a high, shimmering ridge, uses color therapy to surround guests with opulence and a unique ambience. Learning to arrange hues and tones can help you harmonize your environment, change your mood, and beautify your surroundings.

DORAL SPA, MIAMI . . .
The sheer magnificence of this structure includes a curving brick drive beneath a porte cochere, tinkling fountains, and a hush of wealth as pervasive as the warm Florida breeze. A massage like the Doral's can be yours as you follow the author's step-by-step instructions for a full-body massage at home.

MEADOWOOD RESORT AND SPA, NAPA VALLEY . . .
A sanctuary tucked deep in vineyard country, Meadowood specializes in a legendary aromatherapy treatment called the Chardonnay Massage. Now you will learn how to release the powerful healing qualities of grape and other essential oils in your baths, massages, compresses, showers, gargles, and inhalations.

AND OTHER IRRESISTIBLE TREATMENTS. . . .

THE ROYAL TREATMENT

THE
ROYAL
TREATMENT

How You Can Take Home the Pleasures
of the Great Luxury Spas

STEVE CAPELLINI

Illustrations by Michel Porier

A Dell Trade Paperback

A DELL TRADE PAPERBACK

Published by
Dell Publishing
a division of
Bantam Doubleday Dell Publishing Group Inc.
1540 Broadway
New York, New York 10036

Copyright © 1997 by Steven Capellini

The trademark Dell® is registered in the U.S. Patent and Trademark Office.

Book Design by Nancy Field

Library of Congress Cataloging in Publication Data
Capellini, Steve.
    The royal treatment : how you can take home the pleasures of the great luxury spas / by Steve Capellini.
        p.   cm.
    ISBN 0-440-50776-6
    1. Health resorts.   2. Balneology.   3. Massage.   4. Self-care, Health.
5. Relaxation.   6. Rejuvenation.   I. Title.
RA794.C37   1997
613—dc21   97-3174
                                                                   CIP

Printed in the United States of America
Published simultaneously in Canada
December 1997
10 9 8 7 6 5 4 3 2 1
BVG

For my mother and father,
whose encouragement and love have flowed
unceasingly through all the ups and downs

❧ *Acknowledgments* ❧

Scores of people have gone out of their way to support me during this project, and I'd especially like to acknowledge . . .

Agents Elizabeth Pomada and Michael Larsen, who took the years-old dream of this book and made it a reality through their advice, friendship, and hard work. Without them, this book would not exist.

Kathleen Jayes, for her editorial expertise and enthusiasm for the project.

My wife, Atchana, who inspired me all the way, and her mother and sister, Umpun and Lek, who fed me the best Thai food around to keep me going.

Special friend Carole Spellman, who has climbed the ladder beside me, the hardest-working, most-organized, reliable, and trustworthy friend a person could ever enjoy; I'd drive you anywhere.

Brother Jim and sister Tina, for their example of natural, healthy living, and for Lalitha, for her expertise in herbs and healing.

Tara Grodjesk, for her warmth and support and deep knowledge of spa therapy. And her husband, Mark, in loving memorial.

Michel Porier, for his friendship and the beautiful drawings in this book.

Jill Balzer, for posing and for always keeping in touch via the Internet.

Stephanie Gunning, for her belief in the project and her early guidance.

Diane Rose, for her therapy to keep me going during the writing.

Ken Blanchard, for guidance and a new subtitle.

Peter Feibleman, for early recognition.

The spa world is like a big family, and I owe a lot to all of its members. Those whose help was invaluable to this project include:

Cheryl Hartsough, for her spa-camaraderie throughout the years and her expertise in the spa kitchen. Anne Bramham of the Bramham Institute, who added invaluable information about nutrients in spa foods. And Chris Wingate, chef at PGA.

John and Ginny Lopis, teachers and friends, for cultivating a working relationship that allowed me to grow in this industry.

Rainie Giltner, for her help and her specialized seaweed expertise.

John and Laura West, for their friendship, connections, and their ongoing development of spa therapies in the beauty industry.

Robin Zill, Stewart Griffith, and the gang at TouchAmerica, for the fun early days of developing the spa workshop.

For all the marvelous therapists who gave me treatments, advice, encouragement, and who freely shared their knowledge to benefit this book: Kara Mathenian, Wesly Sen, Cristin Coombs, Bryan Porter, Kim Oliver, Marianne Dunn, Clinton and Colleen at the Chopra Center, Theresa, Laura, Larry, and Carlos at the Golden Door, Susan at Enchantment, Maggie at the Phoenician, Chris and Larry at Camelback, Veronica at Sans Souci, Ted Kuminski, Tonya Defriest, Jeanie Wolvers, and Kate Riely.

For the spa owners, managers, and directors who helped me along the way: Maggie Spencer at Sans Souci, Jill Taylor at the Phoenician, Richard and Judy Bird at the Golden Door, Suzzie Bordeaux-Johlfs at Ihilani, Richard Hill, Jim Root, and Mechelle Hill at

Green Valley, Judy Snow at Camelback, Lisa Caruso at PGA, Leslie Wolski and Linda Richie at Sonoma Mission Inn, Trish at Enchantment, Eric and Cathy Chesky at Meadowood, Nancy Cauthorn at Mount View Spa, Joanna Roach at Canyon Ranch in the Berkshires, and Dr. Deepak Chopra, Arielle Ford, Carolyn Rangel, Marcia Ross, Kimberly, and Brent at the Chopra Center.

And for all the people at ISPA who have forged a new professional image in the industry, and who helped me in research.

❦ *Contents* ❧

THE
ROYAL
TREATMENT

YOUR OWN ROYAL TREATMENT

love spas.

I've worked in them for the past twelve years—massaging people with scented oils, spreading warmed fango mud on them, stimulating points on their feet, enveloping them in seaweeds, aiming the jets of high-tech hydrotherapy tubs at their aching muscles, sloughing the rough edges of city life from their bodies with sea salts and aloe, and performing many other treatments as well. I've trained hundreds of other people to do just the same. I've helped to create teams of pleasure experts at some of the most exclusive spas in the country. We've gone through huge shipments of the most expensive ingredients available, and we've mastered the use of the latest cutting-edge equipment. But in the end it's not the fancy ingredients or special equipment that really matters. It's something else.

What is the secret ingredient of any truly superior spa treatment? It's not salt from remote Bulgaria; it's not clay from the Pacific Rim; it's not the precious oil distilled from the fragile petals of a beautiful rose in France.

The secret ingredient is people.

The reason guests leave a weekend's or a week's stay at a spa relaxed, rejuvenated, refreshed, and glowing with health is because they have made the choice to receive, allowing others (the spa experts, therapists, owners, and managers) the opportunity to give. When people visit a spa, they always do so with hope and, whether they know it or not, with the sincere desire to share quality time with other human beings. Nurturing time. Healing time. This book has been created with the sole purpose of introducing you to some new ways in which you can share quality time with the people you care about and with the person you should care about the most—yourself.

When I started in this business in 1984, many people still thought of spas as "fat farms" or as escapes where they could "dry out" after months and years of living a lifestyle that was the opposite of self-loving. My first job as a spa therapist was in one of these "old-fashioned" establishments. Every half hour a gong would sound in the men's locker room, and a squadron of cigar-smoking old men would shuffle down the tiled corridor in paper slippers and clamber up on narrow tables for a rubdown. All the tables were in a big open room, and there was a lot of good-old-boy joking around and crude male-bonding rituals going on. Twenty-five minutes later the full-body massage was over. The men slumped off the tables, shambled back up the corridor, and got dressed again, preparing to head toward the dining room and another meal of tasteless "diet food."

Believe me, things have changed. Today spas mean pleasure and wholeness, beauty and well-being. They are becoming the place to go as an extension of the healthy lifestyles most of us are attempting to create for ourselves at home.

We no longer "escape" to spas. We bring them home with us.

As you turn the pages of this book, you will learn how guests are treated at some of the most fabled spas in the world, such as the Golden Door, the Sonoma Mission Inn, the Phoenician, Canyon Ranch, and Green Valley. The people you'll read about are the working spa experts themselves, people who have made a career out of treating other people like kings and queens. I'll show you how they bring luxury, peace, and bodily harmony into the lives of the people they touch, and then I'll teach you some simple variations of each type of spa treatment that you can easily re-create at home.

You can jump from treatment to treatment and from chapter to chapter in this book. It is recommended, however, that you read Chapters 1 through 3 first, because in them you will find useful information that pertains to all the following chapters. In Chapter 1 you will learn the seven Conscious Pleasure Principles that form the underlying philosophy of the royal treatment. Familiarizing yourself with them will make it possible to fully enjoy all the luxuries that follow. Chapter 2 lists and explains all the equipment you'll need to make your home spa a reality. In Chapter 3 we'll travel to the beautiful Sans Souci spa in Ocho Rios, Jamaica, where we'll learn about body scrubs. In this chapter, my recommendations for your own home spa procedures are explained in greater detail than in subsequent chapters, and they will be used as guidelines to remember when performing the rest of the treatments in the book.

In Chapter 4 you'll meet a native Hawaiian healer on the wild western shore of Oahu to learn about the power of the ocean and hydrotherapy. In Chapter 5 you'll visit the famed Golden Door spa, tucked away in southern California, and see how they use herbs grown right on the property to perform their herbal wrap treatments. Chapter 6 will take you to the Phoenician Spa in fashionable Scottsdale, where you'll learn about a spa-quality facial designed especially for men. Chapter 7 reveals the official uniform for spa goers and home spa stayers alike. In Chapter 8 I tell a story about massaging a very special guest who is an expert in receiving massages; with his help you'll learn how to give and receive a basic full-body spa massage. In the center of the book you'll find the Conscious Pleasure Chart, a valuable tool that will help you choose which treatments to use for various occasions. Chapter 9 will take you to a spa in one of the most dramatic settings in the world—Sedona, Arizona—where you'll learn about special body wraps as they're performed at the Enchantment Resort located in the red-rock canyons. In Chapter 10 you'll hear firsthand from the well-known doctor and author Deepak Chopra as he describes the philosophy of his new Ayurveda spa in La Jolla, California. In Chapter 11 you'll see how guests at the Canyon Ranch spa in the Berkshire Mountains can enjoy the benefits of mineral-rich seaweeds, even though the spa is hundreds of miles from the sea. The top of the head and the tip of the toes are the focus for Chapter 12 at the Green Valley Spa in the desert of southwestern Utah, and I will teach you about hot oil hair packs and spa foot treatments you can do at home. Chapter 13 is a reminder to listen to that inner voice telling you to treat yourself well, even when you're feeling down. In Chapter 14 you'll visit the Meadowood Spa in Napa Valley where they use flower and plant essences for aromatherapy treatments. Chapter 15 will teach you how spas use clays and muds for therapeutic purposes; you'll journey to the Camelback Inn in Phoenix, Arizona, to see how the experts do it. In Chapter 16 you'll meet a renowned spa nutritionist and learn how to begin cooking in the low-fat, high-nutritional manner found in spas. Complete menus for three Spa Days will be included.

When you reach the last chapter, you'll discover that you now have the tools necessary to create a whole Spa Day for yourself and your loved ones whenever you please. Your own home can become a spa sanctuary, and you'll have everything you need to create the ultimate luxurious experience: an explanation of each basic type of spa treatment, information about spa products and supplies, and plenty of detailed instructions. All you have to do is jump in and enjoy.

Let me show you how. . . .

> *"Pleasure is Nature's test, her sign of
> approval. When someone is happy,
> she is in harmony with her environment."*
> —Oscar Wilde

Chapter 1

THE CONSCIOUS
PLEASURE PRINCIPLES

As you open this book, you are putting yourself in a completely new environment: an environment filled with new potential. If you were to take full advantage of every last drop of health consciousness that is available here, you could transform your life for the better in less than one day. If you wholly tap in to these spa therapies, they will bring you to levels of body-awareness that you may not have experienced for a long time—if ever.

What does it take to tap in? It's simple. In fact, it's so simple, it almost always escapes us. In order to receive the full benefit, all you must do is enjoy—fully *consciously* enjoy. Spa treatments present a way to indulge yourself that should ideally be guiltless. There are no laws against them, they harm no one, and they are one hundred percent good for you.

But there's a catch. Almost always, when we attempt to be good to ourselves in such a healthy way, we find a nagging little voice in the back of our heads, saying things like "You don't really deserve this right now. Shouldn't you be putting in that last load of laundry? The kids need you to be spending quality time with them; what are you doing cocooned in herbalized cotton sheets when you could be carpooling to summer gymnastics?" And on and on.

The purpose of this book is to help you help yourself create a new level of nurturing in your life. The time has come for all of us to let go of our old beliefs that luxurious spa treatments are reserved for some privileged upper class, some more leisurely race of humans, always some *other* people who have more time, more money, or more good taste than we do.

Spa treatments today are not just convenient ways to pamper yourself and forget your pains. They are tools to explore higher levels of health. I'm talking about health as a vibrant, dynamic energy in your everyday activities, not just as a lack of disease.

The only way you are going to get this message through to your nervous system is to fully, deeply accept the level of luxurious health these spa treatments will give you *while you are experiencing them*. That means learning how to filter out guilt, filter out self-criticism, and filter out distractions. This may seem like a tall order, but the rewards are tremendous. And the stakes involved are no less than your very Self. You *are* special, on the deepest level, and you've known it all along, ever since earliest childhood, when your little world was the center of the universe and all other people existed simply to please you and to play with you.

You deserve the royal treatment. Give yourself this opportunity.

Today the world is becoming ever more full of the beautiful life-giving sanctuaries known as spas. Soon you may find one in your own town, perhaps in your own neighborhood. Our new modern spas are the focal points we've created to balance out our rapid-paced lives with our need for peace, health, and spiritual fulfillment. As we move into the twenty-first century, spas will become our retreats, sources of wholeness and renewal, feeding our souls as well as our bodies.

As I've traveled the country giving lectures and workshops to people who are opening their own spas, I've been amazed to find interest in every corner of the map. From El Paso, Texas, to Waldoboro, Maine, from Connecticut to Washington State, from Key West to New York City to Kalispell, Montana, and the outer reaches of Michigan's Upper Peninsula, I've found a growing population of knowledgeable, excited professional people dedicating their lives and their livelihoods to the goal of providing their neighbors with these modern-day fountains of youth. You no longer have to travel to the far-flung locales of the famed and fabled spas featured in this book; you can check your local Yellow Pages instead. Or if you'd like, stay in your very own home and create your own sanctuary.

None of these options excludes any of the others. A trip to one of the incredible (and admittedly pricey) destination spas featured in this book can be looked upon as a once-in-a-lifetime reward for hard work well done, or perhaps as a yearly retreat. Day spas closer to home can be utilized on a monthly or weekly basis, for that consistent recharging we all need. And your own home can become a spa that you use every day, even if it's for something as simple as a soak in an aromatherapy bath after a hard day at work.

Products designed for use in spa treatments are evolving every year into increasingly powerful substances. In many of the world's best spas, for example, you won't just find plain old seaweed; you'll find micro-burst, concentrated blends of several of the most powerful sea plants, combined with seawater extracts, pure essential oils gathered from around the world, and absorbent clays from trenches in the ocean floor. Technology combines with nature to create healing. I've listed a variety of these products in Appendix A.

All the pieces of the puzzle have been put in place for you—the best products, excellent treatments from the best spas, and the most highly qualified therapists to teach them to you. Only one thing remains for you to do. It's the simplest thing of all, but in a way it's the hardest. To receive the full benefit from the spa treatments described in the following pages, you'll need to develop and nurture the Conscious Pleasure Principles. These principles have been tried by spa aficionados and health experts the world over. If you follow them one by one, I guarantee that you will enter a new phase in your life. They apply not only to spa treatments but to all activities you do for yourself that are healthy, pleasurable, fun, and uplifting.

The Conscious Pleasure Principles

1. **Preparation:** *Before* heading to a spa, or creating a spa experience in your own environment, consciously choose to set aside ten to twenty minutes to be with yourself in silence. It is a good idea to do this on a regular basis, but it is especially important when you are about to give yourself some healthy pleasure. You'll be amazed at how many tricks your subconscious has to keep you from being completely present and aware when you are about to "indulge yourself." During these minutes scan your body and your mind in great detail. How do you feel? What would you like to change about the way you feel? What feels already strong and healthy? Calmly, and nonjudgmentally, tune in fully to where you are *now.*

2. **Ambience:** Now that you're attuned to yourself, it's time to absorb your surroundings. When you first arrive at a spa, or first step into your spa sanctum at home, stop for a minute and soak in the surroundings. In every case you should find an environment that has been carefully constructed. Pay attention to the details. Spas have a natural aroma created by an abundance of essential oils, sea products, and herbs. Let these scents permeate your every cell. Notice the lighting: dapples of sun falling through trees, a well-placed candle. Take a moment to fully admire the flower arrangements, and listen for the soothing music, both man-made and natural. Are birds speaking to you close by? Is a CD by Enya playing? Really lis-

ten this time. By concentrating on your environment, you can begin to quiet your thoughts.

3. **Greetings:** When you are met by your therapist, your partner, or yourself (in the mirror) before your spa treatment, honor them with a friendly handshake or a slight bow, or perhaps exchange the word *namasté*. Placing your palms together over your heart, utter this simple, sacred word that means "I honor the light within you." Look directly into the eyes before you, especially if they are your own in the mirror. Seek out the warmth and the caring that are surely there in this most nurturing of environments.

4. **Letting Go:** When the treatment begins, gradually and softly let the past go. Start with the past hour, then move to the day; erase the past week, the past month, letting the stress of your whole life slip quietly away. Look within, and let the subtle stresses of guilt, regret, and remorse slip away too. Sages have said it for thousands of years, and they were right: There is only here, only now. Allow this awareness to begin its magical work of healing in your life.

5. **Immersion:** When you are right in the middle of your spa experience, use your breath to tune further and further in to the Present by closely following each inhalation and each exhalation, progressively relaxing each part of your body. As you do so, keep bringing your wandering mind back from the grocery list of your life.

6. **Surrendering to Pleasure:** This is good for you. Honor yourself now for the pleasure you're receiving. Know that it is completely healthy and nurturing, not only for yourself but also for everyone in your life and even strangers you come into contact with. Sometimes, because of the pressures of our modern lifestyles, we find ourselves taking pleasures in ways that hurt other people or ourselves—by overindulging in alcohol, food, or sex, for example. Or by using control or power over others in unhealthy ways. The pleasure we derive from

these activities is always the opposite of nurturing, and it can never be fully conscious. We hide part of ourselves away when we indulge in this manner. But with Conscious Pleasure, we can be fully present and fully enjoying our lives at the same time.

7. **Gratitude:** After the treatment is over, take time to be with yourself again. The best option at this point is to sit outside, near water, under the sky. Of course, if you're at home in Chicago and it's February, perhaps a few minutes bundled up in front of a fireplace or in a cozy bedroom is a better option. Take time to absorb the sensations that your body is now certainly feeling. Let the echoes of pleasure continue to rebound through your inner Self. Notice the increased blood flow, the heightened skin sensitivity, a looseness of limb, a relaxed diaphragm, a rosy, smiling face. See if, just maybe, even though you didn't dare to expect it, you're experiencing something not unlike *ecstasy*. You may surprise yourself.

Now, with these principles to guide you, you are ready to start assembling your very own spa environment. I think you are going to find this an incredibly pleasurable experience, one that will perhaps inspire you to seek out some of the fabulous places and wonderful people that I've had the joy of getting to know over the years. Good luck to you! We're going to get straight away into the treatments themselves, but first a few brief words about practical matters. . . .

Chapter 2

PRACTICAL MATTERS

What You Will Need to
Make Your Home Spa Work

———————

Chances are you have neither an extra room in your house nor an extravagant budget that will allow you to fill it with the sort of equipment found at the spas you'll encounter in this book. If you do have the room and the budget, refer to Chapter 17 for some suggestions. In the meantime, if you are looking for the maximum conscious pleasure for the minimum capital outlay, this chapter will tell you everything you need to know. In order to perform the treatments suggested in the following chapters, you'll need to gather a few inexpensive items and have them on hand.

The Spa Thermal Unit (STU): Otherwise known as a six-pack mini–ice chest or Igloo cooler, the STU is a simple but important part of your home spa setup. It's an insulated container to keep hot towels hot, and the Igloo is the ideal size. Actually, any high-quality cooler or insulated container will do, but make sure it's not too big because if it is, the heat of the towels will dissipate inside. Most spas have heating units called Hot Towel Cabis that cost hundreds of dollars. Yours only has to cost $7.99 at Wal-Mart; in fact, almost all home spa equipment can be found there! I've used them in workshops all across the country, and they work great.

Spa Bowls: Have a quart-sized plastic bowl on hand to hold water, body baths, salts, algaes, and other spa ingredients. You'll find that a simple bowl becomes an indispensable commodity when you set out to perform your own treatments.

Wrapping Sheets: When purifying herbs, emollient creams, and aromatic oils are penetrating your pores, you don't want their effects to be hampered by a low-quality material enveloping your skin. You will need *one* high-quality sheet of "canvas grade" material, either natural muslin or pure unbleached cotton.

Insulating Sheets/Blankets: You'll definitely want to stay warm while cocooned in rich seaweeds or while absorbing pure essential oils. The best choice in warming wraps is, of course, wool. Also highly recommended is a metal-based thermal sheet, often referred to as a Space Blanket. If it was good enough for the NASA astronauts, it's good enough for our home spas. These can be found for ten to twelve dollars in camping stores and some department stores like K mart.

Skin Brush or Loofah: Exfoliation is a key word in the home spa experience, and all of Chapter 3 is devoted to it. Some spa treatments exist solely to exfoliate and slough off dead skin cells, but *every* treatment, including a regular spa massage, is enhanced by a quick whisk-over with a dry skin brush or a loofah. As an added benefit, it's a great stimulation for the lymphatic system.

Towels: Make no mistake about it—spas are towel-intensive environments. The best thing to do is invest in a set just for home spa use. The ideal color is dark green since you may be dealing with seaweed products, muds, and oils. Keep one towel on reserve as your designated "spa towel" to wipe up any mess and clean away excess oil during massage. Many spa therapists keep their spa towel flung over one shoulder or tucked into a belt.

Robes: One thing you'll notice if you visit a number of spas is that people walk around in public areas wearing nothing but bathrobes—fluffy, high-quality sumptuous bathrobes. While this is not an absolutely vital ingredient for a first-class spa, there is definitely something to be said for wandering around in slippers, with the breeze curling around your naked legs. If at all possible, have one hanging on a nearby hook when you are playing spa at home. And this is one area to splurge on; nothing feels quite the same as a high-quality bathrobe. See Chapter 7 for more about robes.

Massage Oil: So many options are available today in massage oils. Most of them are very good. For your home spa purposes, choose a versatile oil that has aromatherapy properties and that is suitable for multiple uses, such as full-body massage, aroma wrap, and foot treatments.

Body Scrubs: Many types are available now, from gentle exfoliants put out by major cosmetic lines to heavy-duty sea salts with big rough crystals.

Herbs: Sachets of healing combinations can be found at most bath and body stores. For information about locating bulk herbs in a variety of formulas, see Chapter 5.

Seaweeds and Muds: These products can be found at many cosmetics counters. Make sure to choose an organic variety, as straight from the source as possible. Suggestions are given in Appendix A.

Thermometer: If you don't have much experience gauging water temperatures by feel, you may want to have an inexpensive pool/Jacuzzi thermometer on hand. Make sure it's the type that can measure temperatures in the upper ranges (above 100 degrees Fahrenheit).

Cotton Pads and Cotton Swabs: For application and removal of just about any product, especially around the face, large circular pads are the best.

In Appendix A you will find a more extensive list of spa products and supplies. With my advice, the Tara Spa Therapies Company has sourced some high-quality natural ingredients and put them together in home spa kits. They range in price from very modest to totally extravagant, for those who want to re-create the whole spa experience at home.

❦ *Chapter 3* ❦

SHE SELLS BODY SCRUBS
BY THE SEASHORE

Sans Souci, Ocho Rios, Jamaica

---

he waves are lapping up against the shore in a syncopated Caribbean rhythm. Your body, reclining upon a low-slung padded bench, soaks up the warmth of the tropical sun. Far in the background, faintly heard, are the strains of a Jamaican calypso band.

You are in a spring-fed grotto, surrounded by hanging ferns and flowering plants. A giant sea turtle named Charlie glides through the crystal-clear waters of the spring. The spa here at the Sans Souci resort is named after this gentle creature. As a guest at Charlie's spa, you are being treated to one of their signature treatments, the Body Scrub, a delight that people travel from all over the world to experience. The skilled Jamaican therapist who led you down into the seaside grotto takes a moment to explain the treatment to you, then begins.

First, you lie facedown on the sun-warmed pads, and a stream of heated water flows over your back. The therapist sprays enough water to leave you moist but not drenched. Then she lifts a bowl of freshly mixed native ingredients in one hand, scoops out some of the contents with her other hand, and proceeds to rub the mixture into your glistening skin. She works vigorously, and you can tell that she has tuned in to the beat of the distant music as her hands glide, stroke, and slough away every last vestige of your former un-scrubbed self. You notice that her hand movements are circular for the most part, swirling around the contours of your body like the natural flow of a river around rocks.

The ingredients in the therapist's hands begin to work their magic. Heavy-grained sea salt, flaky stone-ground island cornmeal, traces of aromatic oils, and a few drops of spring water combine to gently yet thoroughly scrub away dead skin cells, leaving the pores open and clean. Since the skin is the largest organ of the human body and its major vehicle of elimination, it is vital to periodically rid it of the natural buildup of dry peeling cells.

After the therapist has spent about ten minutes scrubbing every last pore in more detail than you thought possible, warm water washes once again over your body. Then suddenly, to your delight, the grotto is filled with the scent of exotic fruits, fresh and heavily ripe, as a mango/papaya body bath is applied liberally to a brand-new piece of natural loofah. The therapist moistens the sponge, then starts in again on your back, taking off any extra corn-meal or salt that might remain. She is careful to move in circular motions once again, you notice. This must be what she was telling you about in her introductory remarks. Every movement of the Body Scrub is an ellipse, making sure not to stretch the delicate collagen of your skin tissues too far in any one direction, avoiding any abrasive pulling. The loofah is rough but not too rough, and you can feel weeks and months of sun damage, wind damage, and neglect being thoroughly banished.

When this phase of the treatment is over, you are asked to turn over onto your back as gently as possible. Now your eyes scan the hints of blue sky through the trellis work of foliage above.

When the cascade of warm water begins to flow over your torso, thighs, and shoulders, you exhale a deep sigh and wonder why you waited so long to treat yourself to this, the first step in your own royal treatment.

After the entire procedure is completed, you are toweled dry, and a creamy emollient lotion is massaged into your skin, first on the front, then the back. You may notice your body drinking in the lotion like never before. After the therapist has finished with this application, you are invited to do perhaps the most challenging task you'll face throughout your entire day—to stand up and leave the grotto. If you're lucky, no appointment will be scheduled directly after yours, and you'll be able to stay for a short while longer. You may drift into the delicious space between sleeping and waking, where you are conscious but there is not one single thought going through your mind, which has become as tranquil, for the moment, as your surroundings.

The Body Scrub is an excellent place to begin your journey of discovery into the realm of spa treatments. It is one of the most basic and rewarding of treatments. Done properly, it will leave your skin cleansed and ready to receive maximum benefit from any of the treatments that follow. Seaweed masks will sink through the pores more quickly. Herbs will be able to penetrate and detoxify that much better. Essential oils will reach the bloodstream with less to impede them. And as a side benefit, you will literally glow. That is why this treatment is often referred to as a Salt Glow or Body Glow. In my spa certification workshops, after I've finished demonstrating the Body Scrub, I always have the students come up to the front of the class. All together, they place their fingers lightly upon the skin of our newly cleansed model, and all together they automatically let out a chorus of oohs and aahs, like spectators at a fireworks display. Not only will your skin glow after this treatment; it will be softer and smoother to the touch than you've ever experienced before. It will cry out to be touched!

If a trip to Jamaica is not in your immediate plans, don't worry. Charlie and the spa will still be there whenever you might have an opportunity to pay a visit. You, however, will not have to depend upon the expertise of a trained spa staff to receive the basic pleasures of a Body Scrub. By the end of this chapter, you are going to know how to perform a Body Scrub right at home. And believe it or not, it is going to feel every bit as good as it would down there in the Caribbean. Well, okay, you may miss the kiss of the tropical breeze or the evocative ping of the steel drums in the distance, but these are details that can be overcome. Keep in mind, especially, the hundreds of dollars that you will be saving by re-creating this spa service in your own home spa. And fasten your sights on the goal of being able to share this treatment with someone you care about. Then just turn up the thermostat, put Bob Marley in the CD player, and close your eyes.

Some variation of the Body Scrub is utilized at practically every major spa in the world today. Many employ salt as the base in a mixture of several ingredients. Others use salt alone. Still others use no salt at all. The specific ingredients you are going to use for your own home Body Scrub are up to you. I am going to offer you a list of possibilities, and from there forward I am going to refer to them, whether used separately or combined, as the "exfoliant."

Exfoliation is the term used to describe any type of treatment that scours dead skin cells from the body. Where did the tradition of exfoliating originate? Why was it started?

The word *exfoliate* is taken from the Latin *exfoliare*. It first appeared in the English language in the year 1612, and it meant "to strip of leaves." The use of exfoliating Body Scrubs, however, extends well back into history. The ancient Egyptians were an extremely beauty-conscious race, and the upper classes spent much of their time tending to their appearance. Besides shaving their heads with bronze razors and wearing wigs, they also developed a large array of cosmetic products. One of these was a type of soda ash that was used to vigorously scrub the skin before rubbing perfumes and ointments in.

The Romans used metal skin scrapers called strigils in their famous public bathhouses. Examples of these early exfoliating tools were found buried in volcanic ash at the baths in Pompeii. In Turkish baths a rough canvas washcloth wielded by a professional masseur did an effective job. For over one thousand years in Finnish saunas people have banished any trace of dead skin by beating themselves all over with the leaves and branches of young birch trees, a procedure that left the skin thoroughly stimulated and quite red as well as clean.

Almost all Native American tribes used some form of ceremonial sweat lodge as part of their culture. This usually included skin cleansing with the use of fir branches, eagle wings, or buffalo tails. They sometimes rubbed their skin with aromatic herbs as well. The Puyallup-Nisqually tribe rubbed themselves with sand after their sweats. The Omaha used grasses. The Mayans and Aztecs used bunches of herbs, and several tribes fabricated special instruments out of animal bones specifically for the purpose of scraping the skin.

In the England of Queen Elizabeth I, as well as in French courts before the Revolution, serious attention was given to achieving that peculiarly pale look of the aristocracy. One way they affected it was to rub a type of white lead into the skin. The ghostly white complexion that ensued distinguished its wearer from the peasantry, who could not afford exfoliation. The peasants had the last laugh, though, and not just in the Revolution. It turned out that the white lead eventually corroded the skin and caused the hair to fall out.

Today, the products used and the methods employed are quite gentle and benign compared with exfoliants past. Comfort is the key at the world's greatest spas, and it should be in your own home spa as well.

Veronica is one of the therapists at Sans Souci who specializes in giving their famous Body Scrub. When asked to describe in her own words what is most important to keep in mind for customer comfort while performing this treatment, she does not hesitate in her response. In a silky singsong voice full of the flavor of Jamaica, she says, "It's the warmth, you know. Without that, no matter how good your technique is, no matter how hard you work or what ingredients you use, the people are just gonna end up complainin', and you don't want that. Luckily for us here, there's a nice warm breeze comin' in off the bay three hundred and sixty-five days a year. And we always make sure to keep our shower water near skin temperature or a little higher, in the upper nineties. For those folks doin' this type of treatment up north, I'd recommend one thing first: Keep that body warm!

"After that, I'd say the most important points to keep in mind are your ingredients—they have to be fresh and aromatic. And of course your attitude. You've got to welcome those people into your special domain and make them feel they're somethin' real special."

Of course, this hospitable attitude directly reflects Conscious Pleasure Principle Number 3—Greetings. Without a true flair for hospitality, any spa would fall far short of its potential. The director at Charlie's spa, Maggie Spencer, echoes her therapists' opinions. In more clipped British tones, she sums up the administering of first-class treatments at any top-notch spa. "It's the caring, really, isn't it?"

This is what the royal treatment is all about.

The question is often asked: "How often should one receive a Body Scrub? Is it safe to do every day?"

Most people who visit a spa receive a Body Scrub only once during their stay, for a particular reason. It should be remembered that the body has its own innate wisdom; if nature did not intend for dead skin cells to remain on its surface, they would fall off by themselves, which in fact they do. A certain amount of dead skin cells remain, however. They actually form the first of the four layers of our epidermis, known as the *stratum corneum*. The dead cells act as a barrier against light and heat energy, and they protect the body from water loss, microorganisms, and many chemicals. So you can see, it would not be beneficial to constantly go scraping all of these cells off in the name of beauty. An occasional sloughing, though—no more than once a week, and especially when combined with other nourishing, replenishing treatments—does wonders and actually helps the skin in its constant process of renewal.

In many large spa facilities an entire room has been constructed solely for the purpose of giving the Body Scrub. The floor and all the walls are covered with tile. In the center of the room usually stands a giant raised stone or ceramic slab upon which the client reclines. A drain is built into the floor, and a shower head attached to a long hose protrudes from one wall. The entire setup is made watertight and mildew proof. Other spas have specially designed "wet tables" that have a drain built right into them.

With the help of certain recent innovations, the Body Scrub can now be given just about anywhere and with a minimum of mess. Some colleagues and I have developed a new system that allows anyone to perform a scrub at home, even in a carpeted room, with no need to worry about water damage or even much cleanup afterward. This is the method I've taught to hundreds of professionals across the country and abroad, and it is what I'm going to teach you in just a moment.

First, let me explain the simple setup you'll need, and a short list of readily available ingredients. You can certainly choose any number of the easy-to-use prepackaged products that are available throughout the beauty industry, and I've listed a few in Appendix A. But everything you need can be found in your kitchen or at the nearest grocery store.

You Will Need:

Three bath towels

Four hand towels

One washcloth

One plastic bowl, twelve-inch diameter, filled with hot water

One loofah sponge

$1/2$ cup exfoliant in small bowl or plastic bottle

Soap/body bath

Spa Thermal Unit (see Chapter 2)

Optional—a Crock-Pot

Exfoliant Recipes

You can head out to any beauty supply store, salon, or well-stocked drugstore and find dozens of options to choose from in the realm of scrubbing agents. Salts from the Dead Sea in Israel are what I personally recommend. They are extremely high in magnesium chloride, potassium chloride, and calcium, three vitally important minerals. The salts can be mixed at a ratio of two tablespoons water per cup and used solo, or you can add grainy flakes of organic cornmeal and a few drops of your favorite aromatherapy oil, as they do at Charlie's spa.

If you can't find Dead Sea salts, any sea salt will do. The heavier the grain, the more intense the exfoliating action will be, which often causes redness, especially on people with light-complected, sensitive skin. The redness—or hyperemia, as therapists call it—is nothing to worry about. If someone is extremely sensitive, though, you'll want to opt for more gentle scrubbing mixtures, and there are plenty of them around today. Most of those commercially available make creative use of naturally occurring substances. One of my favorites is a combination of finely ground almond shells and tiny bits of sea kelp in a cleansing base.

Here are two easy recipes for your own home use. Remember, no matter what you use, it is important that it be kept warm. Nothing's worse than relaxing for a treatment, only to have cold salt slathered on your skin. You can keep your cup or plastic bottle warm by placing it under the hot water faucet before giving the treatment.

Recipe One:

$1/2$ cup sea salt
$1/2$ cup organic cornmeal
3 drops each lavender, chamomile,
    and rosemary essential oils
2 tablespoons spring water

Mix thoroughly into a grainy paste.

Recipe Two:

1 cup sea salt
2 tablespoons almond oil
1 tablespoon water

Mix thoroughly into a paste. Use Dr. Bronner's Peppermint Soap on your loofah as a "body bath."

Setting Up

You can perform most of the steps of this treatment on yourself, although it is a little tricky to exfoliate your own back. Half the pleasure, though, comes from having someone else paying such lavish attention to you. Training a partner for all the spa techniques in this book is highly recommended! Tip: One sure way to get them to give to you is to give to them first.

Before you even bring your partner into the room, spread a large bath towel out on the floor or, if you're lucky enough to have one, on the massage table. A carpeted floor is better than a hard one, and the edge of a bed will work too. Make sure your partner's body fits on the towel; if it does not, overlap two smaller towels slightly and place them end to end so that your partner remains completely on them during the treatment. This way you will avoid any mess later.

Take four hand towels, fold them into quarters, roll them up lengthwise, and dip them in very hot (but not boiling) water. Wring them out, wearing rubber gloves if you have them to protect your hands, and then place them either in the (optional) Crock-Pot or in the Spa Thermal Unit.

One more note about the towels we'll be using. The technical term used by therapists for a hot, wet towel is *fomentation,* which comes from a Latin root meaning "poultice." We needn't concern ourselves with terminology, but several of the treatments in this book are going to use these hot towels, and the techniques for using them described here will be used throughout. It will be best if you practice getting the towels as hot as possible and then storing them in such a way that their heat is maintained for as long as possible. You'd be surprised what a little ice chest (STU) can do in this regard, as long as the towels are sufficiently hot to begin with. Once you have the system down, you'll have a setup that allows you to simulate a hot-water treatment room at a fancy spa with amazing accuracy.

Fill your bowl with hot water, and you're ready to invite your partner in. Of course, you'll want the bedroom or bath or wherever you're giving your Body Scrub to be nice and warm, 80 degrees or higher, as bodies tend to chill quite easily when they're splashed with water, even when the water's warm.

THE BODY SCRUB

Have your partner lie facedown on the bath towel. She can wear a bathing suit, or you can drape her with a towel, or you can do what they do at Charlie's spa in Jamaica—leave your partner *au naturel*! Dip the washcloth in your bowl of hot water, wring it out halfway, and moisten your partner's back and the back of her legs. This step is used in place of the spraying of the shower head at a spa like Charlie's. Next, place a tablespoon-size dollop of your exfoliant in one hand, rub your palms together for a moment, and then apply it to the back with both hands.

The exfoliation stroke is different from a massage stroke in that its purpose is to cleanse the surface of the body, not affect the underlying tissues. Keep your pressure firm but not hard, and make sure to leave your palms and fingers open and flat. Your partner should feel a pleasurable "scrubbing" sensation, but it should never seem abrasive. Movements should always be in a circular direction so as not to pull the delicate skin fibers too far in one direction or another. If you see the skin start to redden a bit, don't be alarmed. As I mentioned earlier, this is completely natural, especially for people with fair complexions. This is simply blood coming to the surface, which is beneficial in cleansing out the capillaries.

This step takes about five minutes. You can swirl your palms around in a rhythmic manner, lulling your partner into Body Scrub bliss. Move slowly down the back and onto the back of the legs. Don't worry about pulling any hair, as the layer of moisture between your hand and your partner's body will make the scrubbing go smoothly. Remember, though, that the purpose of this treatment is to rid the skin of dead cells. A little elbow grease is indicated while performing it. Firm strokes help to circulate the lymph fluids, thus aiding in the elimination of toxins. You can remoisten the skin at any time if you feel a dry, grainy "bunching up" of your exfoliant. Also, add more exfoliant whenever you wish.

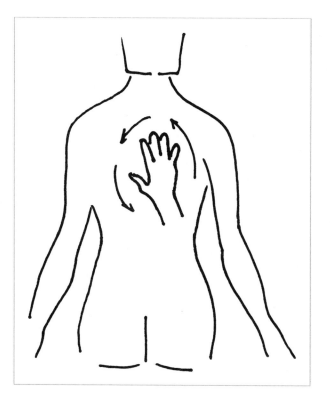

Step 2: The exfoliation stroke—firm but not abrasive.

The next step involves using the first of your preheated towels. When you've finished scrubbing the back, take the towel out of the STU, unfold it, and wave it in the air for a few seconds if it's still too hot. It's usually okay to place the towel on your partner's back a little sooner than you'd think. Your hands are more sensitive than her back, and the extra heat sure feels good.

Run the towel down your partner's back, over the legs, and down to the feet. It is not necessary to wipe off every last grain of your exfoliant now. The very next step is going to take care of that.

This time, dip your loofah sponge into the bowl of hot water, apply a quarter-size patch of body bath to its surface, and begin to scrub. *Note:* Mango or mint body baths are nice for this purpose; see Appendix A for suggestions. This, in effect, is a second skin

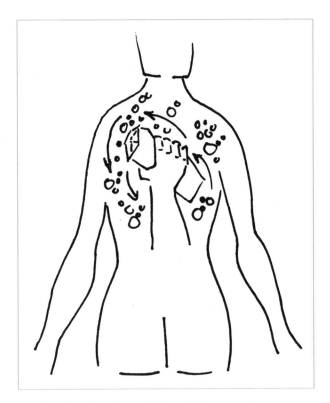

Step 4: Cleansing with the loofah and body bath.

scraping combined with a cleansing. Follow the same rules of pressure and direction you did with the exfoliant, and once again spend about five minutes completing this step on the back and the back of the legs.

Then it's hot towel number 2.

When you've finished with the first two steps, have your partner roll onto her back, and start the process over again, this time beginning at the feet and working your way up. First, moisten the body with the washcloth. Then place some exfoliant in your hand and begin working it in circular motions, first up one leg, then the other. When you've finished there, move to the abdomen, being extra careful, as this is a sensitive area. Women's breasts should usually be avoided because these tissues are too delicate for many exfoliants. Stop when you reach the neck. Gentler products formulated especially for the face are available; most body-scrubbing agents are a little too rough above the neck. Finish off with the arms and hands.

Time for hot towel number 3. Wipe away the exfoliant, starting with the abdomen, as this area feels the most pleasure when presented with such delicious heat.

Move on to dip your loofah in the warm water once again, squeeze some soap onto it, and apply. Always remember to use circles! You can pay special attention to those areas of the body that are normally treated with a pumice stone—elbows and heels especially.

After five minutes use your last hot towel, take off as much of the soap as you can, then pat your partner dry with a clean bath towel.

The final step in the Body Scrub is an application of cream. The richer and more moisturizing it is, the better. This application can last only a few minutes, in which case the whole Body Scrub will be less than thirty minutes long. Or you can make this the beginning of the one-hour full-body Spa Massage, which you're going to learn in Chapter 8. For now, though, just finish the treatment by applying the cream to the front of the body for two minutes. Then have your partner turn over and apply some more cream to her back. When she turns over, you should quickly replace the towel she was lying on with a clean one so that her nice cleanly polished skin doesn't end up in a puddle of sea salt.

What you should have in front of you now is a literally glowing body, not to mention a person who is truly grateful to you and can now almost certainly be counted upon to return the favor someday.

Enjoy!

Step by Step

Start with partner facedown.

1. Moisten back and back of legs.
2. Exfoliate back and back of legs.
3. Rinse with hot towel number 1.
4. Loofah/soap back and back of legs.
5. Rinse with hot towel number 2.
6. Partner turns over onto back.
7. Moisten front of body.
8. Exfoliate front of legs, arms, torso, shoulders.
9. Rinse with hot towel number 3.
10. Loofah/soap front.
11. Rinse with hot towel number 4.
12. Pat dry with a towel.
13. Apply moisturizing cream to front of body.
14. Partner rolls over one last time.
15. Apply moisturizing cream to the back.

The steps for the Body Scrub have been explained in great detail because it is the first treatment in the book, and you are still becoming familiar with your own home spa methods. In subsequent chapters you will build on your knowledge so that you won't need such a detailed explanation.

The combination of these first steps will leave your body perfectly prepared for many of the spa treatments that follow. Or you can make this the last treatment of your own Spa Day. Either way, after you're through, you'll want to run your fingertips over your newly smooth skin again and again—and invite others to do so as well.

"So let man consider of what he was created;
he was created of gushing water."
—*The Koran*

❧ *Chapter 4* ❧

HEALING WATERS

Ihilani Resort, Oahu, Hawaii

O*n the far side of Oahu,* a world away from Diamond Head, Waikiki, and the traffic of Honolulu, you will find a pearl-hued resort shimmering on the edge of a quiet lagoon—a resort called Ihilani. An otherworldly calm pervades the hotel's open-air pavilions, and the mystique of the islands is everywhere.

I arrived one gorgeous afternoon to train the staff at the spa. I had been hired to teach them new techniques in hydrotherapy, but as it turned out, I ended up learning as much from the people I met there as they did from me. After all, the Hawaiian islands have an eight-hundred-year tradition of healing that has been passed down through families from generation to generation.

After being introduced to the group of therapists I was to work with, one of them took me aside. His name is Wesley, and he is a strong and stout native of the islands, with short jet-black hair and a wide smile. "You look like you could use a little island healing yourself, Steve," he told me. "How would you like to receive a special treatment?"

I agreed immediately, and Wesley accompanied me back to my

room. As we strolled through the marble lobby, I couldn't help but notice that he was carrying a thick ten-foot-long wooden pole. Whatever this special treatment was going to be, I hoped it wasn't going to hurt!

In the room Wesley had me lie down on the carpet while he stood above me. First of all, he intoned some sacred syllables in his native tongue. With my eyes closed, I could easily picture myself on these islands hundreds of years earlier, being treated by a great kahuna, or healer. In a clear melodious voice Wesley prayed over me, *"Kou makou makua iloko okalani."* He told me later that this was known as *Pule,* the special prayer that a therapist shares with his patient at the beginning of a traditional Hawaiian healing treatment, in which the therapist and the patient become one with the source of life.

Wesley manipulated the pole along the floor, using it as a balancing device like a gondolier in Venice, and using his feet to open my every joint and press away every last bit of stress I'd carried from the mainland. This, Wesley told me, was traditional Lomi-Lomi massage as practiced by his ancestors for generations, passed down through a series of teachers. For the next hour he continued to sing his soothing songs and to manipulate my body as if it were a musical instrument. All throughout this experience, during which I slipped deeper and deeper into bliss, Wesley told me about his healing tradition and the land from which it sprang.

"We're a people of the water," he said. "My forefathers came from other islands hundreds of miles away from these. Even though the distances were great, we could still communicate. We navigated with the stars and wind. And whenever we met, we passed down these techniques. I myself learned from some elders, Freddie Tira and Margaret Kalehuamakanoelu'ulu'uonapali Ahaulakeali'."

"Whoa, that's quite a mouthful," I said.

He chuckled. "We call them Uncle Freddie and Auntie Margaret for short. It is as if we are one big family across the waters, and this therapy is our language."

Wesley has a very distinct manner of talking, enunciating his words precisely to emphasize his meaning. Lying there, listening to his voice, I could feel the palpable undercurrent of the islands and their people speaking to me. Turning my head to one side, I could see out the sliding-glass door, over the terrace, and out onto the vast moon-sparkling Pacific. I had never seen the ocean in this way before—as a source of life and health.

"The water is where we all come from, isn't it, Wesley?"

"Oh yes, for us the ocean is our Mother, part of Mother Earth."

Mother Earth, Mother Ocean. It was a concept that inspired me. After Wesley left the room that night, I sat on the terrace, wrapped in a warm breeze coming up from the water. Water. The Source. Hydrotherapy. Suddenly everything I had been studying and teaching in spa therapy came together.

When you enter a world-class spa, you enter a world of waters. Cascading waters, swirling waters, soothing, nurturing, curing waters. Modern spas were created in a womb of water. The word *spa* itself comes from the town of Spa in Belgium, where people have flocked for centuries in order to experience the restorative powers of its natural waters. Most of the traditional European spas are places where people go to "take the waters," meaning that they will drink the natural spring waters as well as bathe in them. This is excellent advice for all spa visitors and for everybody who wants to optimize their home spa experience as well. *Drink a lot of fresh, pure water—at least two quarts a day,* in order to wash out impurities and provide a fluid internal environment in which your cells can thrive.

Wesley's healing had sunk into my very core. I woke up the next day feeling a sense of profound well-being and bodily pleasure that seemed to emanate from deep in my joints and viscera. The slight intestinal cramping I'd been experiencing lately was now totally gone, and a lingering pain in my right sciatic nerve had disappeared as well.

Walking over to the spa with a new spring in my step, I found the entire staff there to greet me in what is known as the "wet area." This is the part of a spa that is reserved for treatments focused on water. Molded from white marble and tiles, and highlighted with traces of sea-foam green, the wet area at Ihilani contains a cold plunge, a swirling hot whirlpool, a steam bath, a Swiss shower, and a special high-powered water spray called a Scotch hose. Over a waterproof table a long metal arm extends with five shower heads attached to it—an apparatus known as a Vichy shower. And behind etched-glass doors, in a room all by itself, is the gleaming new state-of-the-art hydrotherapy tub, with seventy-two separate jets and an underwater massage hose that packs enough punch to untie even the most stubborn of muscular knots. I had operated these tubs and taught other therapists how to do the same at some of the most exclusive spas in the country. At twenty thousand dollars apiece, only the most exclusive spas could afford them! I knew how powerfully therapeutic they could be. At the Ihilani, however, they had gone one step further. Seawater was pumped in from the lagoon outside the hotel. A network of pipes conveyed this precious natural ingredient directly into the tub.

Water. The Source. Hydrotherapy.

The key ingredients were all in place. As I stood facing the crowd of therapists gathered around the tub to practice "new" techniques, I remembered Wesley's words. None of this was new. It was the same ancient water language that his people had been praying with and healing with for centuries.

Turning a Bathroom into a Wet Area

You probably already have the ingredients necessary to perform a basic version of the most popular hydrotherapy treatments. Imagine yourself coming home from a particularly hard week at the office on a Friday afternoon and entering your own private hydrotherapy sanctuary, otherwise known as your bathroom! It's easy to do. Remember Conscious Pleasure Principle Number 2—Ambience. It's all a matter of perspective, whether you want to call your bathroom a pleasure palace or a water closet.

I have one special massage client who is an expert at turning her bathroom into a version of a spa's wet area. Whenever Phyllis schedules a massage with me, she spends about half an hour in her bath in preparation for my arrival. She has surrounded the tub with a collection of candles. She has a small tape player perched nearby with soothing music playing. Several bottles and vials of fine bath salts and oils are within reach. And she has a waterproof pillow for her head so she can lean back and relax, looking forward to the pleasure to come.

Any bathroom can be turned into a wet area, regardless of how modest its size or old its fixtures. All you'll need to do is spend some loving attention on detail. Put a lot of thought into your bathroom. Grace it with touches of playfulness, luxury, and warmth. Remember that twenty-nine-dollar crystal water-filled candleholder you saw at the specialty store? Go ahead and splurge. An incense stick unfurling its musky aroma adds mystique. Or light a tiny bundle of dried sage, and use its scent to purify the air.

One word of caution: Water is powerful. Remember, it's the subtle relentless pressure of water that carved out the majesty of the Grand Canyon. Be careful when you indulge yourself with baths. Don't overdo it by staying in the tub for too long. Thirty minutes is a safe maximum, and even less if the water temperature creeps over 100 degrees. Most people can remain comfortable in 104-degree water for fifteen minutes. After that they feel like they have to cool down.

My wife had a firsthand experience of the power of water at one spa we visited. In the morning she received a hydrotherapy tub treatment with concentrated seaweed extracts in the water. Seventy-two jets worked every point of her body while the minerals from the algae were absorbed through her pores. That afternoon we went out for a hike, and she could barely lift one foot in front of the other. Her therapist had told her the treatment might leave her drained, but she hadn't given the warning a second thought. The result: We almost didn't make it up that hill!

HYDROTHERAPY BATH

In order to get most of the benefits of a high-tech spa hydro tub, at a very small fraction of the cost, you'll need to remember one key—the Source. When you soak in your bathtub, remember to add the ingredients that will connect you back with nature. The following bath ideas are taken from three of the other chapters in this book. Keep in mind that these are just a few of the possibilities. There are as many therapeutic bath possibilities as there are natural, health-enhancing products found in the world.

Step by Step

1. First, create the ambience. Surround your tub with candles. Hang a fern or other green growing plant nearby. Import your favorite music into the space via Walkman or CD player, being careful not to get any electrical appliances too close to the water. Tape a card with your favorite affirmations to the mirror over your sink. Hang silken scarves around the room. Have a fresh towel within reach of the tub.

2. While you are filling the tub with hot water (104 degrees Fahrenheit is the maximum), sit on the edge of the tub or the closed commode, and give yourself the ten-minute Foot Treatment detailed in Chapter 12.

3. A minute before the tub is filled, add your special Source ingredient right into the flow from the faucet, allowing it to swirl and mix thoroughly into your bath.

For a bath from the sea	*Add seaweed powder (see Chapter 11)*
For a mud bath	*Add powdered clay (see Chapter 15)*
For an aromatherapy bath	*Add essential oils (see Chapter 14)*

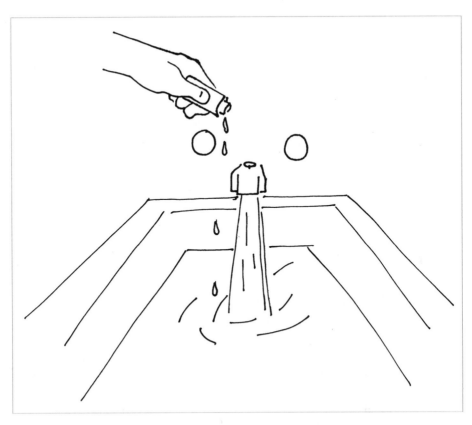

Step 3: Add your Source ingredient to the faucet flow.

4. Step in gingerly, and soak for twenty minutes, remembering to engage all of your senses in the experience. *Breathe* deeply of the healing aromas. *Feel* the waters, bringing them up over your shoulders in cupped palms or with your loofah sponge. Let your eyes linger on the candles and other visual stimuli you've provided.

5. When you've finished, rise slowly and pat yourself dry with a towel, leaving some of the bath's moisture and special ingredients to soak into your skin. This is a perfect time to slip into your robe and do nothing for twenty minutes, to make a cup of tea, or if you're extra lucky, to receive a full one-hour Spa Massage.

Bathing Others—The Sonoma Mission Inn

One of the most sensual things you can do is receive a bath from somebody else. In fact, the bathing and anointing of others has been the essence of spa therapies since Egyptian and Roman times. When it comes right down to it, the best spas are those where they know how to give their customers one heck of a fancy bath. One such spa is the Sonoma Mission Inn, a few hours north of San Francisco, which I visited one day in my quest to learn all I could about hydrotherapy.

Entering the spa grounds through a gate in a pink wall off the side of the highway, I emerged into a softened, time-slowed realm. High-wandering branches of grand old oak trees commingled with towers of fluttering eucalyptus. The hotel itself was pink like the wall, glowing in California afternoon sunlight. Entering the spa building, I felt an opening above my head and looked up to see the ceiling vaulting up like a church nave, filled with skylights. People there, as everywhere in the spa world, were wandering around slowly in bathrobes, talking about the next massage or hydrotherapy treatment they were going to receive.

The Sonoma Mission Inn has been famous for years for the natural hot springs that flow beneath the property, feeding the swimming pool and two communal hot tubs with mineral-laden therapeutic waters. The waters run through the spa's lobby and swirl in pools around every corner.

I was escorted to an inner water chamber where people were steaming and bathing in a coed environment. A small "wet room" adjoins one side of this area, and Kara Mathenia was there preparing a special bathing ritual for me. Kara is one of the spa's lead therapists and an expert at hydrotherapy. When she ushered me into the wet room, she smiled. Her large blue eyes were friendly, and she was wearing a plastic apron over her white therapist's clothes. She looked healthy and strong and relaxed.

"You're going to like this," she said. "It's such a sensual experience. Just lie down on the table there, and we'll get started."

She draped me with a towel as I reclined on a special wet table that is somewhere between a bathtub and a massage table. It has foam padding and sides several inches high. Kara raised the sides up so I was enclosed. Then she began.

After running a natural-bristle brush over my skin, she unhooked from the wall a hose attached to the source of natural waters bubbling and flowing through the Earth below. And she let this water flow out over me onto the table/tub. Next, she ran a mineral-soaked sponge over my skin, cleansing me and rubbing vigorously, obviously enjoying her work.

"This is something you like to do, isn't it?" I asked her.

"I love it because the people I work on love it," Kara says. "It's one of the greatest things in the world, to be bathed by somebody else. Don't you think?"

"Absolutely."

"I offer a similar treatment to my at-home massage customers. I have a whole setup for steam and water and bathing. They love it, like the spa's coming to them!"

Kara continued, using a combination of crystallized salts and mud with the sponge and water to strip away the grime of the world, and using her healthy, uplifting attitude to reaffirm that I was a person worth caring about.

GIVING A BATH

When all of these ingredients are combined—the special spring waters, the luxurious spa, the wet room and wet table, and Kara's attentive touch—what you've got is something greater than the sum of its parts. As people have known for centuries, a bath properly given is a whole lot more than a bath. It's a way of making people feel like royalty.

You Will Need:

A pouring vessel such as a pitcher or large jar

A loofah sponge or natural-bristle brush

Bath salts or oils

Liquid aromatic soap

A soft sponge (natural sea sponges are best)

Step by Step

1. First, as always, prepare your space. Nothing should be over-looked in your quest to create a uniquely comforting environment for your partner. Warm the room. Draw the bath only to half full so that you'll have plenty of space to maneuver. Add the ingredients. Prepare your sponge. And prepare your Self. You will benefit your partner most by being in a calmed, open, giving space, so that he'll automatically feel the impact of Conscious Pleasure Principle Number 3—Greetings.

2. Lead your partner into the inner "chamber" as if this were a very special place, not just a bathroom. The waters you'll be bathing him with may not issue from a thermal spring beneath your house, but they're still life-giving, warm, and nurturing.

3. While your partner is standing on the bath mat before stepping into the tub, use a moistened loofah or a natural-bristle brush to quickly whisk the outer layer of dead skin cells. This is performed on dry skin and should only last a minute. Use long strokes, and move from the extremities back toward the heart.

4. Then have him slide down into the prepared waters. Take your pouring vessel, catch up some of the warmed water from the tub or the faucet, and pour it over your partner's head, his shoulders, and his back, using your other hand to spread the comforting sensation of warmth. If you have a detachable

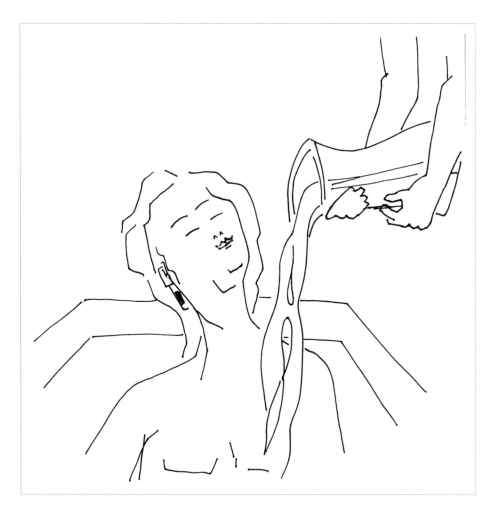

Step 4: Send a cascade of warm water over your partner's body.

shower head on the end of a hose, you can use that instead of a vessel.

5. Apply an aromatic soap to your soft sponge, and begin bathing your partner's back. Dip the sponge in the water frequently, and add more soap if you don't see any suds forming. Run the sponge everywhere, allowing your partner to luxuriate in the fact of another human paying such extravagant at-

tention to him. Have him lie back in the tub, and run the sponge over his chest and abdomen. Have him stick his feet up out of the water, and do his toes. Shampoo his hair if he wants you to.

6. Use the pouring vessel again to wash away the soap. You may also choose to massage his hands or his scalp, rubbing in some jojoba oil, or to simply sit by the side of the tub and talk for a few minutes, enjoying the unhurried time together.

7. Help your partner out of the tub, hand him a towel, and use a towel yourself to help him dry. If there's one thing that feels more luxurious than being bathed, it's being bathed *and* dried by somebody. Total pampering!

8. Rub some moisturizer into his skin and hand him his robe. Chances are you're going to have a very happy man on your hands.

SHARING A BATH

At the Mount View Spa in Calistoga, California, spa director Nancy Cauthorn notes, "More people take hydrotherapy baths together than separately here. It's a big draw for the couples who visit." She showed me into one of the treatment rooms in this famous spa town; the hydro tub there was specially constructed for two people to sit facing each other in the natural thermal waters.

"We normally add a small amount of our organic mud into the waters our customers bathe in," commented Nancy with a smile, "but I don't think it's the mud they're thinking about when they're in here."

It's no secret that sharing a bath inspires intimacy. If there are hydrotherapeutic benefits for your health at the same time, why not indulge right away?

Step by Step

1. Prepare a bath, filling the tub with slightly less water than you would for one person, to avoid overflowing. Add special ingredients like essential oils or mineral salts according to your mood, and light candles and incense. Play some soft music. Try sprinkling rose petals in the bath, or a few gardenia flowers if they're in season. Spread a pathway of towels along the floor, leading up to the entrance to the tub.

2. Wearing your robe, go reclaim your honey from whatever preoccupation he has been caught up in, gently insisting that this is a time for togetherness, a sacred time of communication. Once he enters the sanctum you've created, he'll get the idea.

3. Take turns immersing. Face each other with your legs intertwined. If one partner's back is against a faucet, arrange a couple of towels or a plastic pillow there for comfort.

4. Lean forward, and use scented soap in a soft sponge to lather his shoulders, his chest, and his upper back. Then hand him the sponge and let him do the same for you.

5. If you've finished with a bottle of bath salts or oils, keep the bottle and use it as a pouring vessel. Take turns with your partner filling the bottle, then pouring the warm scented water slowly over every inch of exposed skin—the neck, the shoulder, the knee.

6. Gently cradle his face in your water-smoothed fingers, gaze into his eyes, and tell him how you feel.

7. If any further intimacies develop in the hydrotherapy tub, that is perfectly permissible. It is, in fact, desirable. This is known as "Water Tantra." What better way to take advantage of the pleasures of your home spa environment?

8. After the bath take turns drying each other and spreading some moisturizing lotion into each other's skin. Wrap up in your robes once again, and head together to the kitchen for

an afterbath spa treat like wildberry cheesecake. (See page 199 for the recipe.)

THE COLD PLUNGE

Most of the grander spas have one. They are smaller than whirlpools, and deeper. *Plunge* is just the right word. You'll see people in wet areas standing in front of one, dipping just their toes in, trying to get up the courage. The water temperature is kept to a chilly 60 degrees or below.

The purpose of the Cold Plunge is to close the pores of your skin after they've been opened wide by some form of heat treatment. The result is supreme invigoration.

Try taking a Cold Plunge on those special days when brisk stimulation is your main goal—perhaps before going in for that big job interview. Or when you arrive home from work sluggish and dull but have an important dinner function to attend.

The process is simple. Do what the spa experts do: first heat, then cold. This is also known as "contrast therapy." In Scandinavian countries they plunge from saunas straight into snowbanks!

Step by Step

1. Stand under a steamy hot shower for five minutes.
2. Step out, and wrap yourself tightly in a robe.
3. Fill up the tub with cold water only.
4. Plunge in!

Make it a game to see how long you can stay submerged up to the shoulders. Thirty seconds? Ten seconds? Just two? Most spa guests "pop" back out instantaneously after they've plunged in.

You can then take another steamy hot shower, which should feel twice as delicious this time. You've attained your goal of instantaneous invigoration, and now you're ready for anything.

For a toned-down alternative to the full Cold Plunge, try a "cold foot plunge." The Germans have incorporated this idea into the designs of their city parks. People there take their shoes off and wade into ankle-deep circular walkways filled with frigid water. The effect is rejuvenating, especially if you've been tromping around in high heels shopping all day. It improves the circulation to the entire leg. You can re-create the Germans' idea in your tub; fill it eight inches deep with water as cold as possible (add a few ice cubes if the tap isn't cold enough), then stand in the water or just sit on the edge of the tub with your feet submerged for five minutes. Mountain streams in spring and fall are also great for this purpose.

For more information about hydrotherapy and water treatments in spas:

Croutier, Lyle. *Taking the Waters.* New York: Abbeville Press, 1992.

O'Rourke, Maureen. *Natural Healing with Water, Herbs, and Sunlight.* Miami: Educating Hands Press, 1995.

"Excellent herbs had our fathers of old,
Excellent herbs to ease their pain,
Alexanders and Marigold,
Eyebright, Orris, and Elecampane."
—*Rudyard Kipling*

❦ *Chapter 5* ❧
HERBAL SOLUTIONS
The Golden Door, Escondido, California

A long a quiet inland road in southern California, away from the noise of the big coastal cities, a solitary framed Golden Door stands facing the world. No buildings are visible, just the door. Open the door, descend the hill, and you are living in another world for a little while. The Golden Door spa stands for a level of attention and care and healthy living unsurpassed in the hemisphere.

A Japanese theme pervades the property. Koi slide by in shallow ponds. Doors slide open instead of hinge. Rooms are mingled with tall trees. A rock garden with artistically raked sand patterns sits undisturbed, completely still. People smile quietly.

Most of the time, the Door is a haven for women, but a few times a year the accommodations are reserved for men only. I arrived during such a week.

Walking in a group of men out toward the hiking trails at six o'clock on my first morning there, I passed by the large organic garden that supplies most of the spa's food. The thick vegetal aroma hit my nostrils clean and sharp in the cool morning air: eucalyptus, lemongrass, rosemary, sage. The scent whetted my appetite, but I was soon to learn that the flora provided more than just nutrition. Many of the plants are used in spa treatments as well, and most of the men hiking beside me would soon be absorbing the essences and healing benefits of these very herbs when they received a treatment called the Herbal Wrap.

After several months of the typical highly stressed American male's lifestyle, the state of the physical body can be summed up in one word—*toxic*. In the early days of this century, men would show up at the spas in Hot Springs, Arkansas, and other "spa towns" bleary-eyed on Sunday mornings after their Saturday-night binges. They'd leave it to the masseur and the spa specialist to pound and sweat their sins away.

In the 1990s men are taking care of themselves better on the whole, especially the caliber of men who spend a week at the Golden Door. They are no longer looking for expiation prior to Sunday Mass. They want a regimen that will support their efforts to be healthy all year long. But still, a little detoxification is definitely in order, and nothing fits the bill as well as the classic detoxifying spa treatment, the Herbal Wrap.

Later that afternoon I headed to the spa treatment area where the Golden Door's Herbal Wrap specialist, Carlos, awaited me. He's an impressive-looking man with a full white mustache, and he's been in charge of the men's Herbal Wraps at the Door for over twenty years. As I approached, he already had six steaming-hot herb-infused sheets waiting for me. They had been soaking in a large kettle filled with an herbal solution. Fresh herbs are harvested from the garden, packed into a pouch, and immersed in near-boiling water, making what is essentially a huge vat of tea. The special "herbal sheets" made from pure unbleached muslin are soaked in this solution long enough to absorb the essence of the herbs.

Now Carlos spread the wrung-out sheets on a table, and I started to lie down directly upon them. I was a little too eager, however, and Carlos warned me about the heat. Testing the sheets with his elbow, he gave me the okay after thirty seconds, and I climbed aboard. Soon all six sheets were wrapped around me, and then some rubberized sheets were wrapped around those. To finish the cocooning effect, a wool blanket was pulled over as well.

Immediately I felt my pores, which had already been opened in the steam bath for ten minutes, begin to widen as the heat and herbs took effect. The sensation of heat and enclosure can be overpowering, and Carlos quickly came to my aid with a cold compress for my forehead and face. Each time the heat grew oppressive, he magically appeared with a new compress in hand. For the next twenty minutes I closed my eyes and paid close attention to the tangible sensation of purging through the pores.

One of the earliest practitioners of the Herbal Wrap was Father Sebastian Kneipp, a nineteenth-century Bavarian monk. He used hot herbal essences in towels that he wrapped around patients. Some variation of the Herbal Wrap is used at all the major spas today. The healing properties of plants and herbs are well documented. A large percentage of the drugs prescribed by doctors today are derived from plants. For example, aspirin comes from the willow. Wrapping oneself in herbal essences is one of the most direct routes to receiving their benefits.

The way Herbal Wraps work is quite simple. By raising our core temperature, we fool our bodies into "thinking" they have a fever. The first thing a body does during a fever is to throw off, through sweat, whatever toxins are attacking the system. The herbs used for the solution are chosen for their detoxifying properties, and they aid in the "fever" effect: some draw through the skin, others quicken circulation, others calm the nerves, and others stimulate elimination through the kidneys.

Richard Bird, the spa director at the Golden Door, says, "We choose our herbal mixtures carefully here, changing the blend with the changing seasons because bodies react differently according to the climate. Right now, for summer, we're using rosemary and eucalyptus for their stimulation of the respiratory system, and some lemongrass for a 'sebaceous gland wash.' We pretty much follow the tradition of old Father Kneipp. That's the way the Herbal Wrap was started here by the founders of the spa years ago."

Richard was referring to Edmond and Deborah Szekely, two pioneers in the natural health field who started with nothing over forty years ago and built the Golden Door into the model spa it is today. Now their son Alex helps run the show, and the family is well known for their continuing dedication to healthy lifestyles.

After twenty minutes had passed, Carlos unwrapped me, and I went forth newly cleansed to sit out by the pool, enjoying a cooling breeze coming through the oak trees. My limbs felt like slick sea plants playing in the current of the air, and my whole body glowed from the inside out. An Herbal Wrap expertly administered brings an instant sense of lightness and pleasure. It's best not to dilute that pleasure through exertion or worry for at least half an hour directly following the treatment, which is an ideal time to practice Conscious Pleasure Principle Number 7—Gratitude—to just lie back and enjoy. . . .

In my spa treatment workshops, I teach people how they can re-create an effective and pleasurable Herbal Wrap in their own massage room or even their own living room. This spa treatment needs a little more preparation and equipment than most of the others in this book, but it is still quite simple once you've practiced a bit and mastered the details.

Details are what count in the Herbal Wrap. Heat retention is important, and therefore you have to watch carefully as you follow the wrapping procedure. Also, not just any herbs or wrapping sheets will do. If you grab a bag of Red Zinger tea from the pantry and a mattress-hugging fitted sheet from the linen closet, you're going to end up with a tangled mess of cool sheets and a bewildered partner. Follow the simple guidelines in this section, and you'll surprise yourself at how simple it is to give an effective treatment.

HERBAL WRAP

You Will Need:

- A few ounces of herbs, the fresher the better (although fresh-dried are fine too), preferably from a healthy organic source. Good choices for beginning wraps are:

    1. Chamomile: for soothing the nerves and skin

    2. Ginger root (in small amounts): for stimulating circulation and as a diuretic

    3. Eucalyptus leaves: for the lungs and respiratory system

    4. Rosemary leaves: for the skin and muscles

    5. Clove stems: for soothing aches and pains

    6. Peppermint (in small amounts): for stimulating circulation and soothing nerves

    7. Lemongrass: for its antiseptic properties

- A combination of three or four herbs is good to start with. Try chamomile, lemongrass, and rosemary if they're available. Add peppermint *or* ginger for more stimulation and detoxification.

- A small muslin bag or a piece of cheesecloth in which to tie up the herbs for soaking.

- A high-quality sheet for soaking and wrapping is important. Muslin is the best, but natural unbleached cotton in a thick weave will do nicely as well.

- A pot to heat water in and make the herbal solution.

- A pair of thick rubber gloves, so you don't scald your fingers.

- A rubberized sheet, or Space Blanket, or piece of plastic (like a drop cloth).

- Finally, a wool blanket.

Preparation

First, lay out the wool blanket on the floor or massage table, then the plastic or rubber on top of that. Put an ounce of fresh herbs, or half an ounce of dried herbs, in a piece of cloth or muslin bag, secure the top, and immerse in two gallons of hot water (160–200 degrees) for at least twenty minutes.

Your partner should be either soaking in a hot tub or taking a hot shower during the ten minutes prior to the wrap. If you have a sauna, steam, or Jacuzzi available, that's even better.

You can either soak the herbal sheet in the hot solution or steam it. If you soak it, make extra sure to wear good rubber gloves while wringing it out, or you might burn your fingers. Steaming

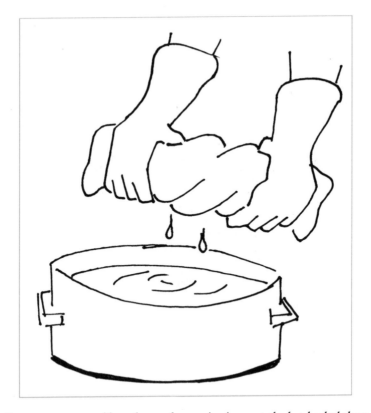

Be sure to wear rubber gloves when wringing out the hot herbal sheet.

the sheet on a rack above the hot solution also works, and it's easier on your fingers, but the sheet doesn't absorb quite as much
herbal essence this way. If you choose to steam the sheet, wet it and
wring it out beforehand, preferably in a cooler herbal solution.

Step by Step

Once your sheet, the wrapping blankets, and your partner are
prepared, you're ready to . . .

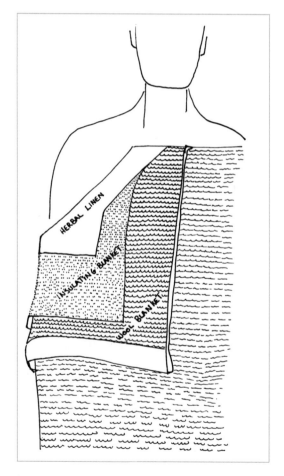

The correct order of the layers for the Herbal Wrap.

1. Open the hot, wrung-out herbal sheet, and spread it on top of the insulation blankets. Try to do this quickly, exposing the open sheet as little as possible to the air, because it will cool off fast, diminishing the effect of the treatment.

2. Have your partner lie down on her back on the hot sheet. She should be wearing as little as possible, in order to absorb the herbs into her skin. Encourage her to climb onto the sheet quickly, even if it feels quite warm, but check to make sure it won't burn her. The trick here is to wring every last drop of water out of the sheet first, because it's the water left inside that will feel too hot, not the fabric itself.

3. Wrap the hot sheet around your partner. If she's prone to claustrophobia, leave her arms outside of the wrap. Make the wrap snug but not suffocatingly close.

4. Immediately begin wrapping the insulating layers around your partner—first the plastic or rubberized sheet, then the wool

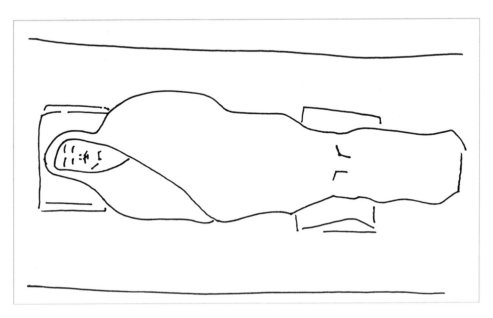

Step 5: Place a pillow under your partner's knees for comfort.

blanket. Place a towel around her face and neck to keep the itchy wool away from sensitive skin.

5. Put a pillow under her knees. As soon as she begins perspiring or when she requests it, offer a cold compress for her forehead. It also feels delicious to have the droplets of perspiration wiped from the face and neck. A sip of room-temperature water can be offered through a straw.

6. Keep her wrapped for twenty minutes, with the lights in the room on low and soothing music playing in the background. Some people will want you to stay with them; others will be fine left alone. Always keep a watchful eye on your partner every few minutes at least. People sometimes feel vulnerable and helpless when wrapped up.

7. After twenty minutes, or whenever she's ready to come out, slowly unwrap your partner. Make sure to have a warm, comfy bathrobe close by because she'll feel chilled no matter how warm the room is when she emerges. Encourage her then to just relax for half an hour if possible, allowing the herbs to air-dry naturally on the skin. Give her a glass of water to drink, and tell her to drink at least three more glasses that day to help the body eliminate toxins and rehydrate.

The Advanced Wrap

If you want to develop more advanced techniques and perform Herbal Wraps very nearly the same as those given in bigger spas, see Appendix A for information about heating units, bulk herbs, and specialty sheets. The following are the points that you'll do differently if you've taken the extra step and purchased these items. This is especially appropriate for people who already do some therapy and want to expand their repertoire.

1. Use a Hydrocollator heating unit, instead of a pot on the stove, to maintain constant appropriate temperature.

2. Instead of steaming, always immerse the sheets directly in the hot herbal solution and then wring them out wearing rubber gloves.

3. Use muslin herbal sheets, high-quality insulation sheets, and 100-percent pure wool blankets.

4. Study herbology, and invent herbal solutions to suit your partner's changing moods and needs.

5. Practice your sheet-wrapping techniques over and over again until you're sure you have a practically airtight seal (without cutting off your partner's circulation).

There are several other spa-oriented treatments you can do with herbs, and they're a lot simpler than the full-fledged Herbal Wrap. Although the wrap is the most deeply detoxifying spa treatment, and my personal favorite, you may not always have time to prepare one. As an alternative, try a quick Herbal Inhalation, Tummy Wrap, or Herbal Bath.

HERBAL INHALATION

Place a pinch of herbs in a porous pouch, and immerse it in steaming hot water in your bathroom sink. Drape a bath towel over the back of your head, then bend over and hold it above the sink in a tent shape. Leaving the hot water running, breathe in the herb-laden steam that floats up to your face from the basin. Your inhalation therapy should last at least ten minutes. Breathe deeply throughout, coughing up any excess phlegm that the steam dislodges. This is especially beneficial if you feel a cold coming on. Eucalyptus is the most common herb used for inhalations because of its healing effects on the respiratory system.

TUMMY WRAP

Heat up a two-gallon pot full of herbal solution, as before. Dip a muslin sheet or a bath towel in, and steep at least five minutes before wringing it out. Remember to wear rubber gloves! When it's cooled sufficiently, wrap the hot towel or sheet around your body from just below the arms down. Then wrap another, dry towel around yourself on top of that. Slip into a warm robe and lie back in a lounge chair or on the sofa to enjoy the warming sensations. Sip a mug of hot tea to enhance the effects.

Because it covers the torso and closely affects the internal organs, this simple wrap has a good many of the detoxifying properties of the full Herbal Wrap. Some people even claim it helps them lose inches, though that's only temporary water loss, and not the intention of this treatment. So don't get too excited if you look thinner for a time directly after the wrap.

HERBAL BATH

Run a hot bath, and place a bag of herbs in the water as it fills up. You can either simmer herbs in a pot, then skim off the liquid and add that to your bath, *or* put your herbs in the small cotton/muslin bag or piece of cheesecloth, and dip that in your tub as it fills up. When it's full, sit down for a soak and enjoy the effects of the herbs you've chosen, whether they be soothing, or invigorating, or tonic, or cleansing, or . . . the list goes on.

For further information about herbs, herb therapy, and healing:

Thomas, Lalitha. *Ten Essential Herbs.* Prescott, Ariz.: Hohm Press, 1994.

To order bulk organic herbs, contact:

Blessed Herbs
Rt. 5, Box 1042
Ava, Mo. 65608
(417) 683-5721

San Francisco Herb Company
250 Fourteenth Street
San Francisco, Calif. 94103
(800) 227-4530

Chapter 6

A FACIAL FOR YOUR MAN

The Phoenician, Scottsdale, Arizona

People who have recently visited spas often seem to shine from within. Something radiates from their skin and draws our attention. In my opinion this effect comes from a combination of three things: (1) greater health and vitality garnered from exercise, fresh air, and detoxifying spa treatments, (2) a new self-confident attitude that comes from being treated like a queen for a week or a day, and (3) freshly glowing, revitalized skin made new and youthful through facials. An extensive program of facials is found today at almost every spa.

When I worked at the Doral Spa in Miami, a woman named Regina was the undisputed master of beauty treatments. She was booked for months in advance, and a facial appointment with her at five o'clock in the afternoon was an extremely prized commodity. What was Regina's secret, and why did people call from all around the world to make sure their time with her was confirmed?

Regina's secret was her warmth and her eccentric Russian character. She has a thick accent and an endearing way of treating people. "Yah yah, I take care of you, no problem," she'd say, patting their shoulder in a comradely fashion. "Come into my room and sit down." She treated everybody the same way, regardless of wealth or social status. A princess felt like a princess in her facial room—and so did every other woman.

Regina was an expert at fulfilling Conscious Pleasure Principle Number 3—Greetings. Through her ability to make each and every person feel welcome the moment they stepped through her treatment room door, she consciously brought her clients an extra level of service and, therefore, pleasure. And that was half of the glow that they left with on their faces. The other half came from receiving a high-quality service well done, plus natural enriching products.

Regina has since moved out of the spa world into her own private business. In search of a facial treatment, I ended up at one of the most polished and glitteringly beautiful spas in America, the Phoenician in Scottsdale, Arizona.

All spa owners and developers know that, upon arrival, their guests will see not only a beautiful building or grounds but a reflection of the beauty they hope to take home with them. At the Phoenician no expense has been spared in creating the most gorgeous reflection possible. The spa is at the base of a multileveled terrace filled with pools. Desert hills rise up in the background, and eternally blue skies open overhead. Descending into the main lobby, you sink into a sea of marble that curls around a front desk, leading directly into the spa's showplace relaxation center, the Meditation Atrium. This space is awash with gentle natural light coming from above through a glass ceiling. Live greenery flourishes in alcoves set aside for recuperation and relaxation. Each private space has a comfortable lounging bed. Water sounds play soothingly in a small fountain.

While waiting in the Atrium for my facialist to appear, an NBA basketball star strolled by in a bathrobe and sat in a nearby alcove. As soon as he sat down, he closed his eyes. This was immediately after the end of the season, and his team had been in the playoffs.

Judging by the relaxed smile on his face, the Meditation Atrium seemed like a perfect place just to "be" for a moment.

I pondered the spa's brochure and found that they have eight different types of facials: the Cleansing Mud Facial, the Gentleman's Facial, the European Facial, the Deep Pore Cleansing Facial, the Collagen Skin Repair Facial, the DNA Pore Minimizing Facial, the Aromatherapy Facial, and the Revitalizing Professional Mask Facial.

I remembered what Laura, a facialist I'd met at the Golden Door, had told me. She's a firm believer in face treatments for men. "Too many men go for a long time without having their skin treated," she said. "They think maybe it's not masculine. But most of the fellows who come here understand how important it is."

The men who go to the Golden Door are certainly the type who know how to take care of themselves. Thinking that maybe there was something to it, I decided to opt for the Gentleman's Facial.

Maggie, the facialist who greeted me there in the Meditation Atrium, agreed with my choice. "Good idea," she said. "If more husbands received facials, I think there would be a lot more happy wives around. Men need to get pampered and look their best too. Come on in."

Maggie's own face was an invitation to her treatment. Her skin glowed with health and vitality, outlined by a thick mane of curly black hair that looked especially impressive on her small frame. She led me away from the Atrium and the front desk, down a hallway, and into a marble room with muted lights. In the middle of the room was a high-tech chair that was reclined so far back, it almost resembled a bed. It was covered with sheets and a cotton blanket that had been turned back, just like a bed also. An array of shining expensive instruments lined one marble wall, their metallic and glassy surfaces gleaming.

Maggie must have read some apprehension on my face. "Don't let the equipment intimidate you," she said. "None of it's painful. Men aren't used to all this stuff, but they always like the treatment once we get started. Just have a seat."

Climbing under the sheets on the chair/bed, I immediately felt relaxed and protected. Maggie's quick skilled hands flickered over her supplies and equipment, fishing out some cotton pads first. These she spritzed with cleanser and used to wipe my face. A piping-hot white towel magically appeared next, lowering down over my face in a cloud of delicious steam. When the towel was removed a minute later, Maggie spent a few minutes looking through a magnifying glass on the end of an extendable arm. She held it over my face while using her fingers to break up oily skin deposits. Then she applied something cool to my face that smelled like Carmen Miranda's headpiece.

"That's a papaya enzyme and pineapple application," she told me. "It's great for cleansing the skin and dissolving impurities because papayas are naturally rich in alpha-hydroxy acids. Just enjoy the aroma, and try to concentrate on the benefits your skin cells are soaking up."

I noticed that Maggie's fingers always moved in the same direction—up. Never did her movements pull the skin around my eyes or mouth in a downward direction. When I asked her about this, she said that it was indeed a conscious technique.

"We always work up," she said. "That's so we're not putting any strain on the delicate collagen tissue of the skin. Gravity is bad enough; we don't want to add any more pulling in the wrong direction. Now I'm going to apply some steam to activate the enzymes."

Reclining in a dimly lit room, with fruit purée being absorbed through my pores and a jet of soothing steam streaming over my face, I found myself in need of Conscious Pleasure Principle Number 4—Letting Go. It's too easy to get caught up in thoughts of other places and other things while the exotic is happening to you right then and there. So I let go of the past and future, concentrating instead on what Maggie was doing.

When she had finished applying the papaya/pineapple mixture and adjusting the steam, Maggie moved to my side, took one of my hands out from under the sheet, and began some massage strokes.

Once the enzymes were properly absorbed, my face was then treated to a seaweed clay mask, which started out green but then gradually turned white as it hardened on my face. After a few minutes Maggie was able to peel it off like a second skin.

She finished the treatment with a flying-fingers massage over my face while spreading some moisturizing cream. Her hands barely seemed to touch me as she flicked and primped the outermost layers of skin into a state of rosy vitality.

Looking at myself in the men's area mirror a few minutes later, I saw a person who looked rich, powerful, and relaxed. Facials seem to bring out the king in a guy.

GENTLEMAN'S FACIAL

Maybe your man doesn't know it yet, but part of him is absolutely craving a royal treatment. He wants to be soothed and taken care of. He wants you to point out how important it is that he look good when he goes out into the world to do whatever it is he does. Through some faulty logic, men sometimes end up thinking that the way their car looks is more important than the way their face does. You can change that.

If you take the time to perform the Gentleman's Facial that I created and am about to describe, your man will definitely love it, even if he thinks you're a little crazy for suggesting it in the first place. A facial is something many men shy away from, but when it's being offered to them by their wives, their fiancées, or their girlfriends, hopefully they'll relax a little and let themselves go.

You Will Need:

Not much is necessary to take your man through a full-fledged facial experience at home:

A comfy chair draped with a sheet

Three hot, moist hand towels in your STU

A bowl of hot water

Some cotton pads

Facial skin toner

Papaya facial blend (see recipe)

Moisturizing cream (see Appendix A)

Seaweed Face Mask (optional)

Papaya Facial Blend

$^1/_4$ cup ripe papaya

2 teaspoons aloe vera gel

2 tablespoons cosmetic clay (from your beauty supply store)

Mix the ingredients in your blender. You can store this mixture for a few days in your refrigerator, but make sure it's warmed up again before you apply it to the sensitive skin of your honey.

Step by Step

1. Don't forget to employ Conscious Pleasure Principle Number 3—Greetings. Warmly welcome your man home from his day. Tell him how special he is and how much he deserves to be treated royally. Help him out of his jacket or shirt. Tell him you have something special planned for him.

2. Lead him to the comfortable chair you've prepared. You can also have him lie down on the edge of the bed or a massage table, on top of a sheet. Place a towel beneath his head to protect the sheets and furniture from stains.

3. Wipe away the day's grime from his face with a cotton pad soaked in a bracing skin toner. Do this for the neck too, and back along the jaw to his ears. This is wonderfully cooling and invigorating.

4. The first of the hot towels from your STU comes out now. Open it up to let the first hit of steam escape, then lower it down onto his face, being careful not to cover his mouth and nose. After a minute pull the towel gently away.

5. Spend a few minutes minutely examining your man's face. Does he have blackheads or whiteheads? If there are any obvious problems you think you can address, go ahead, making sure your hands and nails are extra clean. The most sanitary way to do this is with a piece of tissue paper between your fingers and his face. Remembering to be extremely gentle, squeeze softly from opposite sides of a blackhead, pushing in

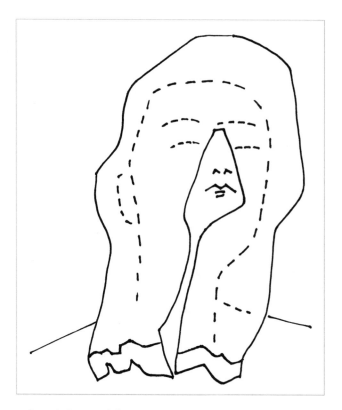

Step 4: Be careful not to cover your partner's mouth or nose with the hot towel.

toward the center. Of course, for the full deep-cleansing of a "real" spa facial, he'll have to visit a professional.

6. Take your (warmed) papaya purée, and spread it out slowly over his face with your fingers, using light massage motions, making sure always to move up toward the top of his head.

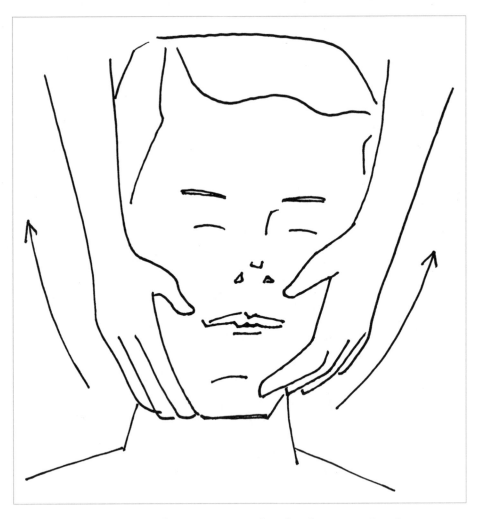

Step 6: Be careful to use an upward stroke when massaging the purée over your partner's face.

You can also apply it to his neck, which feels incredible, and it's good for the sensitive skin there as well.

7. With the papaya blend still on his face, apply hot towel number two. Unfold the towel, and lay the center gently over his forehead. Then circle the ends down around his chin, covering the skin but leaving a little breathing space over the mouth and nose. Let this remain until it is completely cooled off, usually after four or five minutes. Apply the third towel then, to keep his face—and the enzymes in the papaya—warm. It's the heat that activates the enzymes, letting them do their work of activating a deep-cleansing process in the pores.

8. While the hot towels are resting on his face and he is relaxing, take one of his hands at a time, and apply the hand massage strokes listed in Chapter 8. Take your time. Give each hand a full five minutes. Then switch the towel and begin the other hand. Use a rich, soothing cream for the massage.

9. With the last towel that was on his face, carefully wipe up the papaya. You may need an extra towel for this as well.

10. As an option, you may decide to apply a seaweed mask to his face and let it dry. Then either peel or scrub it off, depending on the product. Thicker "rubbery" masks can be peeled off, while thin powder masks can be scrubbed away. (The seaweed listed in Appendix A is of the thinner variety.) Remember to apply only upward strokes and to work gently on the delicate skin of the face. This will add the health-enhancing effects of ingredients found in seaweed, but the papaya facial alone is plenty luxurious enough—don't worry if you haven't gotten your seaweed yet.

11. Using a moisturizing facial cream and slow loving strokes, massage his face. Follow the guidelines for face massage in Chapter 8, remembering to pay attention and not to hurry. How does his jaw feel between your fingertips? What is the texture of his cheeks? Do you feel the beginning of stubble

there after a long day? Glide your fingers over each area, rubbing out care, breathing in relaxation.

12. For the last minute, pull up little portions of his skin between the very tips of your fingers, bringing circulation up to the surface and adding that rosy, refreshed glow to his face. As a final step, when he feels like getting up again, have him look in the mirror for a moment. Is the man he sees now a little different from the one who walked through the door a little while ago? You can congratulate yourself on helping him see the real him.

When he's in the middle of his Gentleman's Facial, remind your man to breathe, enjoying Conscious Pleasure Principle Number 5—Immersion. At first, it may be a strain for him to let himself feel good about the papaya purée spread on his face. It's up to you to remind him that this is his time to forget about everything else, to be taken care of instead of constantly taking care, to let go and let love in.

"I adore simple pleasures. They are
the last refuge of the complex."
—Oscar Wilde

✤ *Chapter 7* ✤
THE SIMPLEST THING

You will undoubtedly notice, if you visit enough spas, that
they are places where bathrobes play a role of major significance.
Walking into almost any spa, you will find dozens of people
wrapped in robes, all of whom seem to be floating on a thin cushion of air, like fluffy terry-cloth ghosts, their slippers slapping lan-
guidly at their heels.

The softer and more luxurious the robe, the higher class the
spa. People in spas take their robes very seriously. Besides workout
clothes—sweats, shorts, and T-shirts—no other item of apparel
gets as much use. At those resorts where only some of the guests
are on the spa program, the lucky ones wear their robes out in public as proud emblems of their favored status. And they wear them
everywhere. You can catch a glimpse of robed and slippered pa-
trons strolling along paths through the Arizona desert, or feasting
on spa cuisine in fancy dining rooms.

Women in fluffy robes sink down into fluffy chairs in warm alcoves waiting for their facialist to appear. Businessmen in robes sit
together in groups, *The Wall Street Journal* upon their laps and the

ball game playing quietly on the locker room TV, waiting for their pedicures and massages.

In the best spas, *everyone* wears a robe—and not just any robe but the *best* robe. What is the reason for this?

Of course, one reason, and perhaps the most fundamental, is a practical one: Going from room to room and treatment to treatment, it is much simpler and smarter to slip a robe on and off instead of an entire set of clothes.

Another reason is the chance it gives the spa to advertise itself on the logo. A good percentage of spa guests end up buying a robe to take home with them.

But there is another, deeper reason behind the tradition of the spa bathrobe. And that reason lies in the very nature of robes themselves. Robes are royal. They invite the wearer to take her time and savor each step she takes, each sensation of sitting down. Each earthbound movement becomes a ballet of sorts, when done in a robe. We have a more immediate and intimate sense of our own bodies with just that one rich layer of cloth encircling our entire form.

High-quality bathrobes are never worn to do work in. They are worn by the people who are currently receiving the fruits of their own labor and also benefiting from the efforts of all the people around them who are working for their pleasure. Robes worn in public confer status.

The world of spas is a world of leisure, and nothing symbolizes this as effectively as the robe. All across the country and throughout the world, wherever spas exist, a world of robes exists with them. This world is populated by a citizenry all intent on the same objectives—indulgence, luxury, the fulfillment of themselves and their dreams.

Unmistakably, the worldwide uniform for this set is the robe.

Purchase *the most luxurious bathrobe* you can find anywhere for any price. Make this purchase an extravagant one. Don't hold back because of practical concerns. This is the one instance in which to let yourself (and thoughts of your bank book) go.

Go for the best. If a famous designer's logo ends up over your left breast, so be it. Or better yet, if you can find someone to do it for you, have your own name sewn into the rich downy material, or create a logo for your own home spa. Joan's Day Spa or The Smith Family Spa are a couple of examples.

Next—and this is just as important as the quality of the robe itself—*sit around in the robe,* preferably propped up against half a dozen warm overstuffed pillows in your bed, and *do absolutely nothing* for at least fifteen minutes. Don't read. Don't think about what you have to do tomorrow. Don't make that important phone call. Just sit. Cast yourself fully into the sensations your body is absorbing. Play the part of the spoiled mistress who has no pressing engagements other than pleasing herself in the moment. At the very most, if you just can't seem to sit still and revel in your good fortune, you may polish your nails. But that's all.

A good time to do this is while the bathtub is filling with steamy hot water. Set the faucet to fill slowly so you'll have plenty of time to do that most basic of all spa activities, *lounge around.*

As an alternative to lounging around, try *walking slowly with no purpose.* With your robe cinched snugly about your waist, perhaps cradling a large mug of cocoa or hot coffee, take a leisurely tour of your home. Include the backyard if the weather's nice enough. And if you're feeling particularly adventurous, amble out into the front yard toward the street. Don't even try to pretend to pick up the newspaper. Just walk. Stand out on the sidewalk for a minute, surveying the neighborhood as if it were all your private domain. Then leisurely turn and stroll back toward the front door. Any neighbors who happen to spot you will immediately get the feeling that they are missing something you have and they do not.

Your magic, priceless possession? *Free time.* Just a few moments of it are as rare as pure gold. Stroll about in a truly first-rate bathrobe for a bit, and you'll take a large first step toward entering the special space that most experienced spa goers know so well—the land of timeless ease and relaxation.

This is just about the simplest thing you can do to re-create part of the true spa experience. But as we all know, sometimes the simplest things are the best.

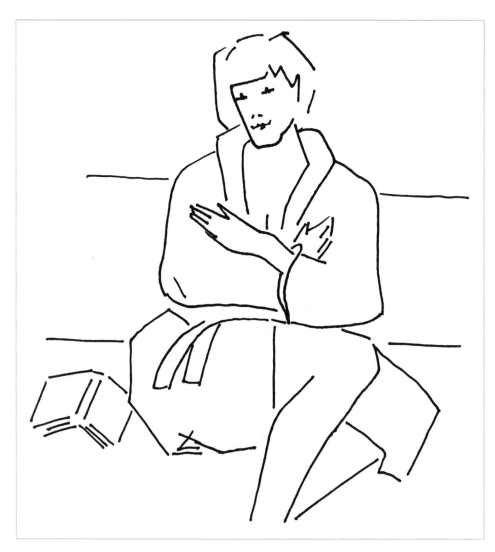

"Touch is a very powerful message. It is very honest. People know immediately when you touch them if you care about them."

—Ken Blanchard,
The One Minute Manager

❦ Chapter 8 ❦

THE ULTIMATE TREAT: A ONE-HOUR FULL-BODY SPA MASSAGE

Doral Spa, Miami, Florida

It was after eight o'clock at night when I got the call, and I was already at home after a full day of giving treatments at the Doral Spa in Miami. Could I come do a late-night massage for a very special guest? My body was definitely in need of rest, but when I heard the name of the guest, I found myself unable to refuse.

Well after eleven P.M. I drove up to the front of the stately property. Even though I'd been employed there for over two years, the sheer magnificence of the structure never ceased to impress me each time I passed the guardhouse and followed the curving brick drive up beneath the porte cochere. An Italian-tile roof soared up to a pyramidal tip where the resort's banner flew in a gold stanchion. I parked my car and headed in past lightly tinkling fountains. Bronzed Tuscan figures poured water from upturned vessels over

The Royal Treatment

73

each other. The hush of wealth pervaded the entryway. Lush palms lined the front walk, their fronds completely still in the warm Florida night. As I entered, I turned left toward the guest rooms instead of my usual right toward the spa building itself.

A portable massage table was waiting for me, along with two very excited co-workers. "I can't believe you get to massage him," said our spa nutritionist. "I met him earlier tonight, and he's just as funny in person as he is in the movies or on TV."

Hoisting the massage table over my right shoulder by its strap, I walked quickly down the long hallway, upholstered with a thickly woven beige carpet without a speck of dirt on it. The guest rooms always left me speechless. Several of them had been created especially for the resort by a renowned Milanese designer. Each suite was different, patterned after the charms of a particular Italian city. I was headed for the Rome suite.

I knocked on the door. A woman in her seventies, wearing a floor-length cream-colored robe, opened the door and let me in. Busying myself in the suite's antechamber, I prepared the table, linens, and oil. Then I had a few seconds to take a deep breath and focus myself. I had to admit I was excited.

A moment later, one of the world's most beloved entertainers and comedians entered the room wrapped in a white towel. He was in his eighties at the time, and even late at night, after a banquet performance, he was still ready with a quip for his youthful massage therapist. "Aye," he exclaimed, reaching around and touching his lower back with one hand, "I've got a pain as big as Saddam in there."

This was during the Gulf War, and his acute political awareness extended even to the massage table. With his wife hovering nearby, he climbed up onto the table and quickly gave me a list of everything I should do for the next hour. He was an expert at receiving massage, having outlived three personal massage therapists. He told me he'd gotten a massage almost every day of his life for the past fifty years, and he credited his health and longevity in large part to this fact.

We were ready to begin. I placed a little oil in one palm, then rubbed my hands together, warming them up. I took another deep breath. He stopped talking and prepared himself with a deep breath also. I poised my hands inches from his back. His wife floated out of the room. We were alone. It was completely silent. Just my hands and his back.

Now what? What could I do? How could I possibly make this man feel as good in just one hour as he had made me and countless other people feel for so many years with his inspiration, humor, and love?

You might think it was easy for me, that I was trained, that any therapist would know what to do automatically. But the truth is that every massage is a new experience. At least every great massage is, and I specialize in giving great massages. As the lead therapist at the Doral, I had been written about in magazines and newspapers and had even been on TV. What made my massages so sought after? One thing—caring.

With total concentration, I cared about this special man's back, about relaxing his muscles and taking away his stress. Then, slowly, I lowered my hands onto his body and began once more the dance of therapy and communication that every hour-long session of massage involves.

Over my years at the spa, I had the chance to share this form of therapy and communication with several other special people. One of our country's most renowned sex therapists ended up on my table one morning, and the humorous, uplifting stories she told me during that hour left me feeling as though I were the one who had received the therapy instead of her.

Another person who impressed me was the star of a major morning TV show. She spent a week at the spa filming a series of shows, and during that time she came down with a nasty cold. Deciding to practice the medicine she was preaching to her millions of viewers, she received a series of spa treatments and massages to help her body rest and fight off the infection. When she entered my massage room, I felt the powerful presence of a woman who was taking charge of her own life and her own health. Her example has helped shape the lives of Americans in every walk of life, and as she lay there quietly on the massage table, absorbing healing energy into her own body, I knew that it would be communicated to people everywhere.

These days professional massage therapists study for many months and pass a battery of tests before working in a spa, but the essence of their effectiveness still remains that quality of caring and sharing, which is something you can nurture for yourself at home too.

So how to begin? I'm sure many of you have experimented with oils and some well-intentioned maneuvers in the past. That is definitely a first step in the right direction. What I'd like to add are some tips gleaned from fourteen years of experience, thousands of massages given, and the know-how of the hundreds of excellent therapists with whom I've had the opportunity to work. Massage people working in spas have to be experts at packing all their best moves into fifty or sixty minutes. They have to adapt quickly to a wide variety of body types and psychological types. And they have to learn how to draw upon deep reserves of caring when faced with long days of work and many clients.

What follows is a distillation of the best oils, the finest moves, and the most beneficial images and visualizations to go with them. As long as you follow these guidelines gently and pay attention to your partner's reactions, you'll run no risk of stretching somebody too far or rubbing too hard. Let your caring be your guide.

Oils

Most of the better massage oils used in spas are created using aromatherapy properties, as described in Chapter 14. One of my favorite scents for the full-hour massage is a mixture of lavender and sage. It's cleansing, detoxifying, and relaxing all at once. This is the blend used for "a love wrap" in Chapter 9. Many of the premixed blends found in health food stores and body product emporiums are wonderful, but make sure not to scrimp in this one vital area, because in terms of fine oils, what you pay for is what you get. Invest in a high-quality oil, use it sparingly (as I'll describe in a moment), and enjoy it for a long time. Hint: Try to find the type of bottle that has a slow-flow cap. Large openings tend to encourage overuse, spills, and oily sheets.

Movements

A good massage therapist blends all of his movements together so that the massage feels like one flowing dance. However, you'll want to learn the basic steps of that flow first. Eventually you will become comfortable enough to leave them behind and embark on a new creative flow of your own. Until you reach that point, use the following seven maneuvers. They come from the traditional type of massage offered at every spa today, called Swedish massage (so named because of the Swedish doctor who developed it), and they are in the basic repertoire of all first-rate spa therapists.

Long strokes—These are long flowing movements meant to soothe. Use your palms either separately or together to glide gently over the skin. *Effects:* Spreads the massage oil, warms up the muscles, and lets your partner's body get accustomed to your touch.

Kneading—Roll and press your partner's muscles in both hands exactly as if they were dough and you were kneading a loaf of bread. *Effects:* Brings circulation into the area, helps unwind taut muscles and fascia, and is deeply relaxing.

Pinpoint pressure—When you find points that are painful to the touch, "bunched up," knotted, or especially hard, use your thumb or forefinger to apply pressure directly on the area. Press just hard enough that the muscles hear the message to release, but not hard enough to hurt. Hold for a count of ten while your partner

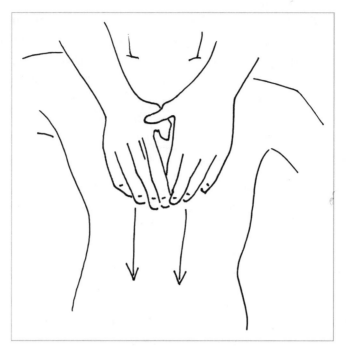

Long strokes

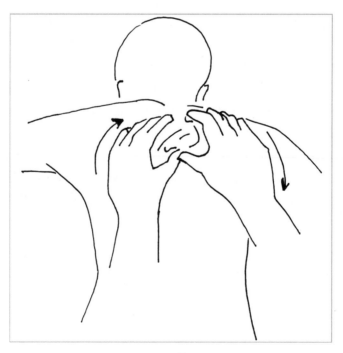

Kneading

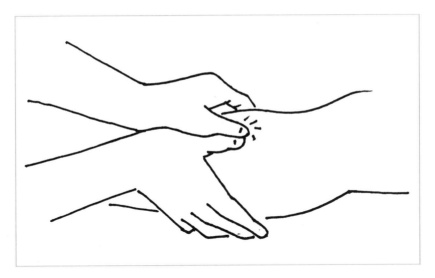

Pinpoint pressure

breathes in deeply. Then relax your pressure at the same time your partner exhales. *Effects:* Gives muscle spasms and tense spots relief by gradually helping them to release chronic holding patterns.

Deep friction—With the thumb or fingertips, make small circles, ranging in size from a quarter to a teacup, pressing just below the surface of the skin onto the muscles below. Also, instead of circles, at times you can make short (just a few inches long) straight lines at this level of pressure. *Effects:* Soothes deeper areas in muscles made tight by exercise and everyday stress.

Skin rolling—This one is often easier without oil. Pinch a fold of skin up between your fingers, then walk your fingers forward, maintaining the roll while moving. It's tricky at first, but keep trying. Most people love it. *Effects:* Lifts skin away from underlying tissues, aiding in superficial circulation; improves skin tone.

Percussion—With loose wrists and the hands in either a cupped or a "karate chop" position, gently and rhythmically tap upon your partner's body. *Effects:* "Wakes up" the body, brings a tingling feeling and increased vitality.

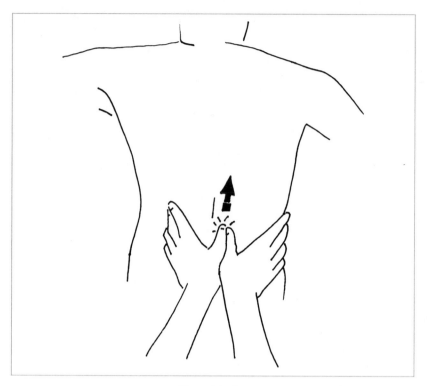

Deep friction

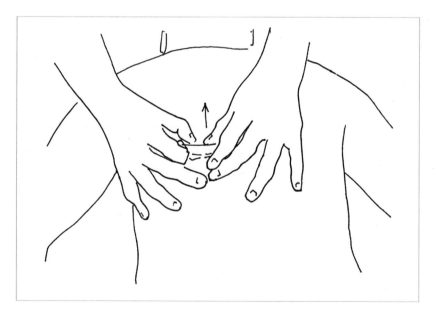

Skin rolling

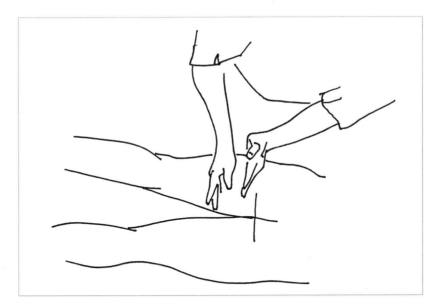

Percussion

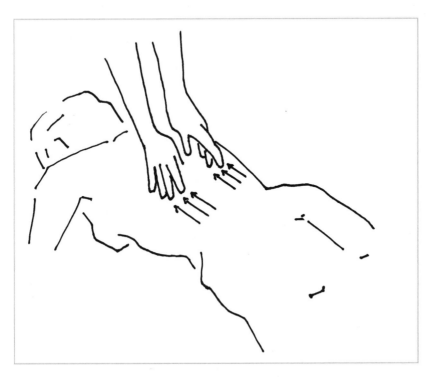

Fingertip brushing

Fingertip brushing—This is done usually at the close of each section of the full-body massage. Using just the tips of the fingers, with very light pressure, gently graze the surface of the skin that you have just worked on. The sensation is delicious. *Effects:* Calms and soothes the nervous system. Relaxes extrastimulated muscles directly after deeper massage.

Body Mechanics

Therapists who work in spas, giving seven, eight, or sometimes more treatments per day, know that they have to move their bodies in very specific ways in order not to wear themselves out early or perhaps even cause themselves injury. You won't be putting in a full day's worth of treatments on your partner, but it is still important for you to maintain good alignment, balance, and movement—a combination of ingredients known collectively as body mechanics.

Whenever possible, keep your shoulder, elbow, and wrist in a straight line so you're not putting too much stress on the joints. Thumbs are especially prone to overextension during massage work; be careful not to press too hard when the thumb is stretched out.

As you move around your partner, remember to keep realigning your body with hers, putting yourself in the most comfortable position that still gives you enough maneuverability to work.

General Rules Regarding Massage

1. When using oil, pour it first out onto your palm before applying it on your partner. This warms the oil slightly, avoiding any shock of coolness on the skin.

2. Deeper strokes that affect blood flow should be directed toward the heart.

3. Be careful with your nails. If possible, clip or file them down before giving a massage. If you need to keep them long, use the pressure of your finger pads instead of the very tips.

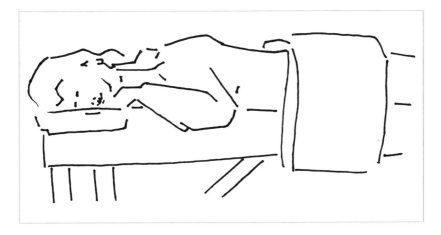

Use draping to show respect for your partner's modesty.

4. The Spa Massage is one hour long, on average. Of course, there is no need to limit yourself if you're feeling inspired, but here are some guidelines if you'd like to follow a typical spa therapist's routine: the back, twenty minutes; the back of the legs, five minutes each; the feet and front of each leg, five minutes each; the chest and abdomen, five minutes; the arms, five minutes each; the head, neck, and shoulders, five minutes. This will give you a total of sixty minutes.

5. Chances are, you already know your partner quite well and are comfortable with him. Even so, during a massage many people like to feel the sense of protection that comes from proper *draping*. Draping is the use of sheets or towels to cover your partner for reasons of modesty. Always respect your partner's needs in this area, keeping them as covered as they like.

THE SPA MASSAGE

Atmosphere

First, find a suitable location. For those of you who already have a massage table, you probably know the best area in your home to set it up; a bedroom or unused guest room is usually ideal, as each affords a feeling of privacy and peace. Because most people do not have a table made especially for massage, the routine that follows takes place on a bed or on pillows and cushions that have been arranged on the floor. Arrange the area, making sure it is even and comfortable. On top of the cushions, pillows, or mattress, spread a bath sheet or beach towel to catch any excess oil.

When you enter a great therapist's room at a top spa, you'll feel something special in the air. It's a mood or vibration. Usually you'll notice some signs that they've paid a great deal of attention to the tiniest details. You can strive for this in your own space as well.

Do yourself the honor of lighting a candle, or ten. Candles have been used in sanctuaries and temples for centuries to induce a feeling of contemplative calm. These days you can find candles in the shape of pyramids with semiprecious stones inside, candles in the shape of goddesses and nymphs, and candles rich with the scent of your favorite essential oil. If candles are not available, place a scarf or towel over the lamp and create your own muted lighting. Experiment! Be careful not to let the scarf get too close to the light bulb, though.

Now head for the CD or tape player. Music in the background is ideal for massage, but make sure not to overpower your partner with an excess of syrupy flutes or New Age piano. At times something slightly more upbeat than usual is a pleasant surprise during massage. Once at the Doral Spa, during a lazy afternoon, I put some light reggae on the central speaker system that ran into all twenty-six massage rooms. Turning the volume down low, I braced myself for a revolt by guests and therapists alike, but as it turned out, I had no reason to worry. The massage staff loved it, and five of the guests actually asked if the reggae tapes were available for purchase!

Beginning the Massage

With your partner facedown first, kneel at her side in a comfortable position, your bottle of oil close at hand. Close your eyes for a moment, centering yourself with a few deep breaths. Then remembering Conscious Pleasure Principle Number 3, Greetings, open your eyes and give your partner a smile. She is prone, vulnerable, and ready to receive with both her body and her mind. Look into her eyes, sharing your healthy, pleasure-giving intentions.

Pouring a quarter-size puddle of oil in the palm of your hand, rub both hands together until they are well covered. Turn the palms over, holding them over your partner's back about eight inches above the shoulder blades. Keep them there until you can begin to feel the heat rising from her skin. Think for a moment about your intention to care for and nurture your partner. Send your hands the message that they can do the job as well as anyone; they can heal, nurture, and make whole.

Then, ever so softly, bring your hands into contact with her back, not seeking to do anything at first. Just let your hands and her back *be* together for a minute. Now you can begin. . . .

The Back

1. Let your first movements be *long strokes*. With your fingers pointing down, gently glide toward the base of your partner's spine. Then turn your fingers out, curving them around her hips as you slide back up the ribs to start at the top again.

2. Positioning yourself at your partner's side, reach across her body using *long strokes*, then lift up on your return, stretching and opening the ribs and sides.

3. Locate the long band of muscle running along either side of the spine. Starting at the base, work your way up, applying *deep friction* circles. Whenever you run into an area that feels extra tight or hard, stop there for a minute and apply slow, gradual *pinpoint pressure*.

4. Using your palms, press against the bone at the base of the spine. Then use both thumbs to make *deep friction* circles all across this area.

5. Little by little, widen these circles out until you are applying *deep friction* to the entire hip area and the tops of the buttocks.

6. Applying a wide grip, start *kneading* the upper hips and onto the side and all over the lower back.

7. Switching positions somewhat, face up toward your partner's head and reach up to grasp the big muscles atop each shoulder. Taking one at a time in both hands, apply *kneading* for a few minutes. This is the area most typically bombarded by everyday stresses.

8. Grasping a small roll of skin between the thumbs and forefingers of both hands, begin walking up from the base of the back toward the neck. You can start near the spine, then move out toward the sides. Some people absolutely love this. Others would just as soon have you skip it. You'll have to ask your partner. If too much oil is on the back already to get a grip, you can wipe the excess away with a towel.

9. We all hold loads of tension around and beneath our shoulder blades. By placing your partner's elbow farther out to the side and tucking her hand up against her rib cage, you'll find the shoulder blade lifting away from the tissue below. Now you can reach into the hidden muscles close to the spine, applying short straight lines of *deep friction* and *pinpoint pressure*.

10. If this massage is intended to be more invigorating than relaxing, try a minute or two of *percussion* at the end of the back segment. Taking your cupped palms and using them like soft fleshy hammers, tap all over your partner's back, thumping out the last vestiges of tension. Be careful not to tap directly over the spine. If it is meant to be more of a soothing, relaxing massage, finish the back with *fingertip brushing*.

The Backs of the Legs

1. Moving farther down along your partner's side, begin with a series of *long strokes* up one leg from the ankles to the thighs. This is a good time to apply oil once again, especially if body hair is present. Be careful around the backs of the knees; make sure not to apply too much pressure, because this area is very sensitive on many people.

2. Do some *deep friction* circles around the anklebones and along the Achilles tendon.

3. Apply some sumptuous *kneading* all over the calves, a progressively stronger movement that starts out light and ends by squeezing out every last drop of tightness in these well-used muscles.

4. Make three *deep friction* lines with your thumbs, straight up the belly of the calf muscle from the ankle, one in the middle and one on each side.

5. Grasp the whole lower leg, encircling it with both hands at the base. Then squeeze while pushing slowly up toward the knee.

6. Do some more *long strokes* on the upper legs for a moment. Then *knead* there as well, taking extra care with the inner thighs, which may be more sensitive.

7. Making a loose fist, graze your knuckles over the long hamstring muscles, lighter at first and then digging in, until you are performing a *deep friction* with your knuckles. You can switch and use your fingertips for this too.

8. *Knead* into the buttocks, and then look for the tight spots that are sure to be there. Apply *pinpoint pressure* to those areas, and you'll most likely observe a big "release" in these muscles, which are the largest in the body. They will quiver, then suddenly feel looser beneath your finger.

9. Do some *percussion* with your hands in the karate position all over the buttocks, hamstrings, and calves.

10. Finish with *fingertip brushing* from the top of the leg down.

11. Repeat on the other leg. Then in a quiet voice, ask your partner to slowly roll over onto her back now.

The Feet and Front of the Legs*

1. Holding one heel in each hand, start with a gentle pull of both legs, holding the stretch for twenty seconds. This is called *traction*. It opens the joints and relaxes the muscles around them.

2. Begin with the right foot, cradling it gently in both hands. No need at first to do anything. In fact, one of the things most therapists learn in school is that sometimes the touch is more important than the technique. One exercise we do is to just

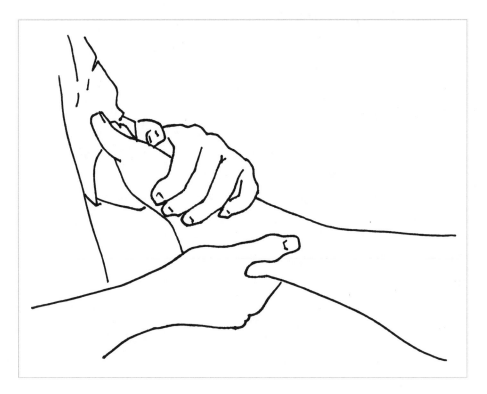

Step 2: Remember that sometimes touch is more important than technique.

*Note: A more comprehensive foot massage routine is offered in Chapter 12.

hold one foot for ten minutes, then feel the difference afterward between that foot and the other. Try this for just one minute. It's amazing! Then, using both thumbs, spread open the sole from the balls to the heels.

3. Making a fist, rock your knuckles over the whole sole, back and forth.

4. Rub and pull gently on each toe, paying special attention to the large toe.

5. Do *deep friction* upon the top of the foot and the sides of the ankles in tiny dime-size circles.

6. Apply oil with *long strokes* to the front of the legs, then spend a minute doing *deep friction* lines alongside the shin bone.

7. Make *deep friction* circles around the sides of the knees, being careful to avoid the kneecap.

8. After a few preliminary *long strokes* on the thighs, moving upward from the knees to the hips, begin *kneading* the inner, outer, and upper thigh muscles.

9. After they are thoroughly warmed up, do a few strokes of *deep friction* lines upward along the thigh muscles. You can have your partner bend her hip and knee and fold the knee out to the side while working the inner thigh.

10. Finish with some light *percussion* on the thighs and then some *fingertip brushing* from the hips down to the toes.

11. Repeat on the other leg.

The Chest and Abdomen

1. Remember that, for most people, the abdomen is the most sensitive and vulnerable area of the body. Positioned at your partner's side once again, start with light *long strokes* from one side of the rib cage to the other, then turn these strokes gradually into circles, always moving clockwise, which is the direction of digestion.

2. Making quarter-size circles from the right hip up to the ribs, across the base of the ribs, then down the right side, do *deep friction*. Then smooth the circles out into lines.

3. Very gently apply *pinpoint pressure* into the soft area between the belly button and the ribs.

4. Reaching across the body, pull up on the waist area while you apply *kneading*.

5. Positioned above your partner's head, do some *long strokes* out from the breastbone to the sides over the chest muscles. On women, this stroke follows a line above the breasts.

6. *Knead* the chest muscles, one in each hand, by grasping them right where the arm connects to the body.

7. Do some *deep friction* circles all down alongside the breastbone.

8. Finish with *fingertip brushing* from the top of the chest, down over the breastbone, and out into large curves on the abdomen.

The Arms

1. Sit facing your partner's head, at her side, and take her hand into yours. After applying some massage oil in *long strokes* from the hands up to the shoulders, spread open her fingers, and slip yours between them, causing a delicious stretch all through the webbing of the hand.

2. Apply *pinpoint pressure* to her palm with your thumbs while you are still spreading the fingers open.

3. Gently pull on each finger, making microscopic *deep friction* circles around each knuckle.

4. Holding your partner's wrist firmly in both hands, shake it up and down for three seconds, loosening the joint. Then make small *deep friction* circles over the back of the wrist.

5. Apply *kneading* to the forearm muscles.

6. Then, holding the wrist in your left hand, stroke up toward the elbow with your right thumb, making *deep friction* lines.

7. Gently lift your partner's arm over her head. Supporting her elbow with your right hand, use firm *long strokes* over the back of her upper arm with your left hand, contouring your palm around the belly of her muscle. Imagine your fingers pushing out old blood, allowing a free flowing of new circulation to reach the area. The return stroke toward the elbow should be softer and more superficial. Repeat this move four or five times. When you feel comfortable, you can try alternating the supporting hand on the elbow, stroking down first on the triceps, then on the biceps. Only a small amount of oil is needed to help with this stroke, as there is normally little body hair and a smooth surface on the upper arm.

8. Lay your partner's arm back down at her side, then use soft *fingertip brushing* from the ends of her fingers all the way up to her shoulders.

9. Repeat on the other arm.

The Head, Neck, and Shoulders

1. Seated above your partner's head, apply one last warmed palm's worth of oil by using a graceful curving *long stroke* that starts at the top of the chest, curls over the shoulders, then sneaks up the back of the neck, ending at the ears.

2. Turning the head alternately to one side and then the other, use the tips of your index and middle fingers to do some *deep friction* lines that run down from the base of the skull to the shoulders. If you find any place that is particularly tight, apply some *pinpoint pressure* while asking your partner to breathe deeply and relax.

3. Make minuscule *deep friction* circles all around the base of the head where it joins the neck.

4. Cradling your partner's head in one hand, *knead* the back of her neck with the other hand.

5. Let your partner's head come gently to rest again, and then begin to touch her face using tiny *skin rolling* movements, starting on the chin and moving up along the jaw.

6. Using firm *fingertip brushing,* stroke out from the center of the face toward the ears, starting at the mouth and moving up to the forehead.

7. Apply a full minute of *deep friction* circles around and around the top of the head and down along the ears, thoroughly banishing any last thoughts about keeping a prim and proper hairdo intact.

8. Finish the massage by cradling your partner's head in both palms for a minute, sending healing thoughts and warmth to every part of her being. Then gently move yourself forward and run your fingers one last time over her face, neck, shoulders, arms, torso, hips, legs, and feet, using *fingertip brushing* while moving down along her body.

SELF-MASSAGE

You might find it challenging at times to inspire a partner to share the joys of massage with you, especially if that partner is going to be on the giving end. When nobody else is around, or when you are the only one in just the right mood, learn to feel good about sharing massage with that most pamperable of all persons—yourself.

In order to successfully complete a self-massage, you'll need to follow the Conscious Pleasure Principles as much as or perhaps even more than during a massage with your partner. Being good to yourself, by yourself, just for you, can be one of the most challenging things of all to accomplish.

The easiest place to give yourself a massage is in a chair. Sit comfortably upright but not stiff. A well-padded chair is best, with a high back for support. Wear some loose shorts and something sleeveless on top.

As you sit down in your chair to begin the self-massage, remember to breathe! Practice Conscious Pleasure Principle Number 4—Letting Go. When no one else is there to help get you in the mood, you need to take charge of your own relaxation. Try to tune out the cares and worries of the day, along with its sounds. A quiet room where you'll be alone for twenty minutes is best. Have your bottle of massage oil close at hand, but you won't need it for the first couple of movements.

Step by Step

1. Letting your head loll loosely forward, raise your hands up and find those perennial knots on the top of your shoulders and the back of your neck. Apply some *kneading* and *deep friction*. Use your left hand to massage the right shoulder, and the right to massage your left, while you turn your head from side to side, stretching out the muscles as you massage them. Finish this move by rolling your head slowly in circles, first in one direction, then in the other.

2. Using all of your fingers, apply some *deep friction* circles to your entire scalp area. This is not a time to worry about your coif; let it go, and thoroughly get into the sensations.

3. Continue your finger circles down onto your forehead and your face. The big muscles at the hinge of your jawbone especially like firm pressure. Then pinch down along the edge of your jaw to your chin on both sides, using a mini–*skin rolling* technique. End by smoothing your palms across your face from the center-line outward, then applying some *fingertip brushing*.

4. With the thumb of one hand, apply *pinpoint pressure* into the palm of the other, searching for tender spots and circling into the sensation. Then *knead* the entire palm and the back

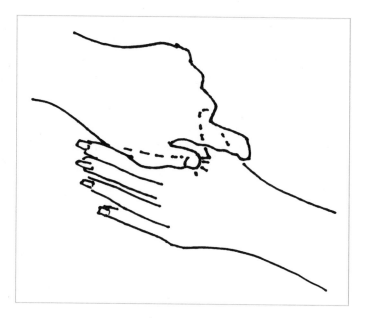

Step 4: Apply pinpoint pressure to the webbing
between thumb and index finger.

of the hand, paying special attention to the webbing between the thumb and index finger. Grasping this area and squeezing tightly with the end of your thumb and forefinger can sometimes help relieve headaches by allowing energy, or *chi,* to flow freely once again. A powerful shiatsu point is located here; stimulation of this point frees the energy. Finish the hand by squeezing from the base to the tip of each finger.

5. Use *kneading* to inch your way up the forearm, stopping and digging in with *pinpoint pressure* wherever you find sore areas. When you reach the elbow, switch to the inside of the arm and *knead* the biceps. Knead back down, and then switch to the outside to *knead* the triceps.

6. When you reach the shoulder, use *deep friction* circles up onto the top of the chest and all the way to the breastbone.

7. Repeat steps 4, 5, and 6 on the opposite arm.

8. Lean forward slightly in your chair. Reaching around to your lower back with both hands, use your fingertips to do *deep friction* circles on the tailbone and surrounding area. Then open the palms up, and *knead* your hips and the upper, outer edges of your tush.

9. Now you can grab your bottle of massage oil and pour a little into one palm. Rub the palms together for heat, then run them both up and down the top of one thigh repeatedly in *long strokes.*

10. Apply some *percussion* to the thigh.

11. Bend the leg you're working on, and bring the ankle up to rest on your opposite knee. Then thoroughly *knead* the calf muscle, working down onto the Achilles tendon.

12. When you reach the foot, grasp it with your fingers on top and squeeze your thumbs out toward the sides, spreading the sole. Rock your knuckles back and forth over the sole, and when you find any sore spots, apply *pinpoint pressure.* Use *deep friction* circles around the ankles and lines along the tops of the feet, between the bones. Then squeeze each toe from the base to the tip. If you feel inspired and would like to spend a little more time on your feet, follow the guidelines in Chapter 12 for the ten-point Foot Massage.

13. Repeat steps 9 to 12 on the other leg.

When you're finishing the massage on your feet, it's a very good time to remember Conscious Pleasure Principle Number 6— Surrender to Pleasure. Admit to yourself that it's completely all right to make yourself feel good this way, that by relaxing yourself, you're doing the others in your life a favor as well. In fact, everyone in your life who truly cares about you will applaud your efforts to be good to yourself. They will support you in creating the time to take care of yourself.

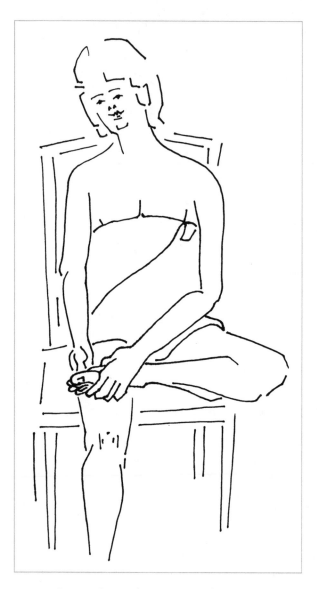

Surrender to pleasure—you deserve it.

The Conscious Pleasure Chart

This chart will allow you to cross-reference all of the treatments suggested in this book. There's a column for six treatment categories you'll want to address, and each row shows how the particular treatment affects them.

Treatment	Relaxation/ Stress Relief	Togetherness/ Communication	Detoxification/ Cleansing	Consciousness/ Spirituality	Luxury/ Pampering	Health and Fitness
Body Scrub (p. 24)	Very relaxing, as long as you remember to keep your partner warm!	Nothing makes for togetherness like scrubbing someone you love.	Through the process of exfoliation, the body is detoxified, at least on a superficial level.		Someone else runs warm water over you and cleans you with soapy sponges; can't get better!	Healthy, clean skin means a healthy body.
Hydrotherapy Bath (p. 36)	Great for letting go of the day's cares.		When the right ingredients are added to the bath, it can be quite purging.		The silken texture of a bath oil or mineral bath salt can be deeply sensual.	Powerful effects: be aware of how it can drain you. Schedule exercise accordingly.

Treatment	Relaxation/ Stress Relief	Togetherness/ Communication	Detoxification/ Cleansing	Consciousness/ Spirituality	Luxury/ Pampering	Health and Fitness
Giving a Bath (p. 39)	Absolutely wonderful relaxation for the receiver. Also, a type of languid sensual pleasure for the giver.	The dance of giving and receiving is particularly rich here, like a princess and her consort.	Can be remineralizing or detoxifying, depending on the products used in bath.		One of the most luxurious experiences in the world is to be bathed by another.	Good postexercise. Improves overall hygiene.
Sharing a Bath (p. 42)	Especially if both partners have been working or under lots of stress, this will definitely melt it away.	Probably the best thing you could do for intimacy. Add eye contact and candlelight, and you've got it made!	If natural spa products are added to the bath, therapy can be achieved, but it's not your aim here.	If you breathe together and focus on your lover's presence, it's known as Tantra—sensual delight.	Use big sponges and lots of rich bath oils to create a luxurious double-giving, double-receiving treatment.	
Cold Plunge (p. 44)	Only for the extremely hardy.		Repeated use strengthens the immune system.	Some monks take cold baths at 4:30 A.M. If you try it, you're sure to have a "spiritual experience."		The most physically stimulating and invigorating of treatments. Great for circulation.

Herbal Wrap (p. 51)	Some people "zone out" during an Herbal Wrap and find it relaxing. Others not so much.	Mild togetherness. Can be fun if you prepare it together and take turns wrapping each other.	Excellent. The best way to purge your body through the pores. A spa detox mainstay for years.	Some people report "leaving their bodies behind" when wrapped in the heavy herbal sheet.	Can be luxurious, but be careful about claustrophobia—leave the arms out in that case.	Good for those quitting smoking, caffeine, etc.
Herbal Inhalation (p. 56)	Just the act of breathing deeply is enough to bring relaxation usually. The herbs are a great excuse.		Purges the respiratory system and helps the body get rid of built-up mucus.			By clearing out the lungs, you're preparing the body for many types of exertion.
Tummy Wrap (p. 57)	Sit wrapped up in your hot sheets and a robe for 20 minutes, and you'll find relaxation.	You can do this wrap alone, but sharing it can make it more enjoyable.	Great detoxifier. Especially good for the internal organs if you have a mild upset inside.		Not as luxurious as the full-body wrap.	Water weight can be lost quite easily, but it's only temporary.

Treatment	Relaxation/ Stress Relief	Togetherness/ Communication	Detoxification/ Cleansing	Consciousness/ Spirituality	Luxury/ Pampering	Health and Fitness
Herbal Bath (p. 57)	Very de-stressing to soak in any bath; add cleansing, invigorating herbs, and you double the effect.		Milder detoxifying properties than the wrap, but still perceptible.		Surrounded by candles and music, with the rich aromatic herbs rising from the tub, this can be luxury.	Allow plenty of time before physical exertion after the bath.
Gentleman's Facial (p. 63)	Taken slow and easy, this is a most relaxing treatment.	One of the best ways for a woman to say "I love you."	Cleansing the pores and adding the enzymatic activity of papaya makes this a facial detox.		Men aren't as accustomed to the pampering, and they find out they love it!	
Spa Massage (p. 83)	For centuries, this has been the treatment of choice. Recommended by physicians and therapists for stress relief.	A nonverbal dialogue is built between two people in a good massage. Good way to expand communication.	Flushes lactic acid from the system and increases circulation.	A great massage is definitely a spiritual experience.	This is what guests come to spas for. Quite often, the height of first-class care.	Hippocates, father of modern medicine, prescribed massage. Great for recovery and athletic preparation.

Self-Massage (p. 92)	A good way to unwind after a long day.		Not quite as effective as massage from a partner.	Pay loving attention to yourself, and you are halfway to nirvana.		Some of the benefits of partner massage.
The Loving Touch (p. 111)	When both parties are tuned to the same frequency of touch, there is no more room for stress or worry.	The experience of going beyond words and communicating through touch can be astounding.	You may experience some cleansing on the psychic level when you focus on somebody in this way.	This is the foundation for the consciousness in all the other treatments. Touch with your spirit.	Once again, the amount of attention paid by one person to another is the foundation for all luxury.	When you "tune in," sometimes amazing healing can take place without your even knowing how.
A Love Wrap (p. 113)	Quite a good stress buster.	Wonderful, healing time to spend with another person. Wrapping adds to a sense of security.	The dry wrap brings a mild detoxification.	Stay focused, and this simple treatment can transport you and a partner into another world.	The slower, the better, and this treatment can become a great luxury.	Mildly toning for the muscles.

Treatment	Relaxation/ Stress Relief	Togetherness/ Communication	Detoxification/ Cleansing	Consciousness/ Spirituality	Luxury/ Pampering	Health and Fitness
Home Journey for Yourself (p. 122)	By taking time for yourself in this way, stress levels go way down.		Mildly cleansing through initial exfoliation.		A great treat for one!	The self-massage in this treatment is especially beneficial for the circulation.
Home Journey for Your Partner (p. 124)	Excellent.	Good ritualistic way to spend time together.	This is part of the *panchakarma* program of cleansing in Ayurvedic medicine.	Done in the same silent, reverent spirit of the Chopra Center, this can be greatly uplifting.	Highly luxurious while being therapeutic at the same time.	Through cleansing and anointing, the body is rejuvenated.
Double Touch (p. 126)	This may be more invigorating than stress relieving.	Three-way communication is good for family/close friends.		Under the right circumstances, three minds-bodies joining for peace and pleasure—great!	The ultimate. Just remember Conscious Pleasure Principle 6. You've got to surrender!	
Meditation (p. 128)	Practiced on a daily basis, meditation is the bedrock of any true stress-relief program.	Through meditation, we often learn more about ourselves, which we can then share with others.	Purging the mind of old thought habits is perhaps the truest detoxification.	Excellent. The straightest path to communion with your inner Self.		When the mind and spirit are calm and healthy, the body soon follows.

The Seaweed Wrap (p. 138)	Wrapped up in a warm cocoon with sea minerals soaking into your pores, you'll definitely relax.	Applying seaweed paste to a partner sometimes promotes a playful sense of togetherness.	Some detox in this wrap. Not as strong as the clay wrap. But the remineralizing makes up for that.	Can be very luxurious if the room is warm and the wrap is comfortable.	Remineralization is the key here to benefiting overall health. Great for the skin too.
Seaweed Self-Wrap (p. 141)	Give yourself enough time to perform this simple self-wrap, and you're sure to de-stress.		This is just as detoxifying as the regular wrap, but be sure seaweed covers as much skin as possible.	With nobody else to bother you, you can stay wrapped as long as you like—and luxuriate.	This is a good way to repair the skin and entire body after long spells spent out in the sun.
Seaweed Bath (p. 142)	One of the best ways to unwind in the tub is with the cleansing, revitalizing effects of sea plants.		Helps in detoxification on a cellular level.	Treating yourself to a bath with the added rejuvenating effects of sea minerals is a true luxury.	Some rejuvenating benefits, but be careful about overexertion after a seaweed soak; it's draining.

Treatment	Relaxation/ Stress Relief	Togetherness/ Communication	Detoxification/ Cleansing	Consciousness/ Spirituality	Luxury/ Pampering	Health and Fitness
Seaweed Face Mask (p. 143)	Nothing fights stress better than looking at yourself in the mirror and finding a green face staring back.		All the nourishing qualities of seaweed work wonders, especially on the delicate tissues of the face.		This is luxurious as long as essential oils are included in the seaweed blend to mask the scent.	
Hot Oil Hair Pack (p. 148)	Good for relaxation. Treating the head seems to benefit the mind too.	A nice way to care for one another. Conducive to long bonding sessions afterward.			Extremely luxurious; reminds people of how Cleopatra must have felt.	Shiny, lustrous hair is usually a sign of inner health as well.
Foot Treatment (p. 155)	Somewhat relaxing, but you really need a partner for full relaxation. Definitely a stress buster.		Stimulation of the reflex points of the feet is tonifying for the whole body.			Great health benefits, even when you're treating your own feet.

Partner's Foot Treatment (p. 156)	Very relaxing and stress reducing. Offering up your feet is like offering up all your cares and worries.	The humble and giving act of massaging a partner's feet will do wonders for most relationships.	Reflexology stimulates the body to eliminate, most noticeably through the kidneys, bladder, and intestines.	The height of luxury. A good time for Conscious Pleasure Principle 6—Surrender to pleasure.	A tonic for the entire body, simply by treating the feet. Further reading in reflexology is highly recommended.
Right Books (p. 157)	For relaxation, nothing beats curling up with a good book and a hot cup of tea.	The communication is with the authors—often excellent, uplifting companions.	Escaping with a good book often brings us back to the world renewed and ready to help again.	An absolutely essential component to anybody's spiritual path is the wisdom contained in books.	It's often the inspiration found in books that puts us on the path to greater fitness.
Color Therapy (p. 159)	By creating a conscious color environment, you lower your levels of environmental stress.	Bring someone else into the creation of your colored world, and it becomes a shared vision.	Purge old blah colors from your life, and you'll feel much better.	To have a color scheme in your life that you've created adds consciousness and is uplifting.	Silken scarves and other rich hints of color add a touch of luxury to any room.

Treatment	Relaxation/ Stress Relief	Togetherness/ Communication	Detoxification/ Cleansing	Consciousness/ Spirituality	Luxury/ Pampering	Health and Fitness
The Emergency Jacuzzi (p. 163)	The very best, because you're consciously taking yourself from high stress back down to low.		You will definitely feel renewed if you make the effort to pull yourself out of a negative space.	One of the most conscious things you can do—halt negativity in the present moment.	Being good to yourself, when you need it most, is the most luxurious thing you can do.	Lowered stress means longer life.
Aromatherapy Massage (p. 171)	The power of essential oils combined with massage induces deep relaxation. Certain oils reduce stress.	By sharing the process of choosing favorite oils, partners spend quality time together.	Specific oils have a deep purging effect and should be used sparingly. Refer to the chart in Chapter 14.	Oils such as sandalwood and cedar can have an uplifting effect on the psyche.	Since antiquity, royalty have depended upon essential oils for their daily dose of luxury.	Various oil blends including eucalyptus, rosemary, and others are great for sports applications.
Aromatherapy Applications (p. 173)	Depending upon the oils chosen, all the applications can be very stress relieving.		When used advisedly in soaks, wraps, and inhalations, certain oils are great for detox.	Depending upon the oil, any of these applications can be calming, which is an aid in meditation.	All the applications are slightly luxurious, but none so much as the aromatherapy massage.	Baths and compresses with the right oils can aid in recovery after exercise.

Mud or Clay Wrap (p. 180)	Mildly relaxing.	More detoxifying than mud or clay bath because mud dries on the skin, drawing out impurities.	This can be luxurious, if you don't mind that "organic" sensation of mud on the skin.
Mud Face Pack (p. 182)	You'll feel the edges of your mouth slowly turn up into a smile when you treat yourself to this mask.	Detoxing to the pores of the face, especially a clay mask, which draws out impurities.	
Mud or Clay Bath (p. 183)	Very relaxing, especially with a candle or two nearby, and perhaps a good book.	Sends minerals from pure earth sources directly into your pores.	Like all baths taken in leisure and aimed to improve health—a luxury. A good way to soothe tired muscles after exertion. Before exercise, be aware—the soak may leave you drained.

Treatment	Relaxation/ Stress Relief	Togetherness/ Communication	Detoxification/ Cleansing	Consciousness/ Spirituality	Luxury/ Pampering	Health and Fitness
Sport Fango (p. 184)	Relieves the stress placed on specific muscles through deep-acting therapeutic properties.	A definite fun-time to be had by giver and re-ceiver as your childlike enjoy-ment comes out.	Mud will bring new minerals to the area; clay will help draw out swelling that tends to occur.			Great for minor aches and pains after workouts.
Mud Hand Pack (p. 185)	For taking the stress off tired, sore, over-worked hands, nothing beats this one.		Purges the joints, bringing renewal and relief.			This can help you avoid some serious compli-cations of repeti-tive-stress syndrome.
Mud or Clay Foot Soak (p. 185)	Great for relax-ation if you really take the time to kick back and enjoy this one.		A clay soak can be purifying by drawing toxins out through the soles.		Even when it's you soaking your own feet, you'll feel well treated.	Great after exer-tions involving your feet, such as hiking, walk-ing, climbing, etc.

Chapter 9

A LOVE WRAP

Enchantment Resort, Sedona, Arizona

The walls of the canyon surrounding Enchantment are filled with the spirits of Sinagua Indians. When you stand on the grounds of this resort in Sedona, Arizona, you can feel their presence. When you walk down to Enchantment Circle at the end of the property in Boynton Canyon, you feel literally surrounded by them. Up on the ridges of the red-rock cliffs, you can still see their cave dwellings, the ruins of their rocky homes. Ancient voices, ancient lives, crowding all around.

The resort of Enchantment itself blends into the cliffs that envelop it. Adobe-style *casitas* curve up into the lips of the canyon, and right in the center, across a raised walkway from the lobby, is the spa. People gather there for treatments and for refuge. As I arrived at the spa desk, one of the managers from the resort was standing in the foyer, head tilted back, breathing in deeply. "I always stop to smell the eucalyptus," she said, and then she headed back to work.

Trish, the spa director behind the desk, said that was typical.

"The rest of the resort comes to be with us because we're different," she asserted, "more laid back and peaceful. Yesterday one of the women from sales and marketing came up just to sit in the women's locker room for a while and chill out."

That's true about most spas—they're havens. And the one at Enchantment is a special retreat, secluded as it is all alone in a canyon several miles from the small town of Sedona, nestled in territory considered sacred by the Indians. When you enter its sacred space, you suspect something extraordinary might happen. And that's exactly what did happen to me when I received a treatment called the Pueblo People Wrap.

Of course, the Pueblo people are the Indians who inhabit the Southwest. Native Americans all throughout North America used rudimentary forms of hydrotherapy in their daily lives. Traces of early sweat lodges have been found in many areas, and frequent use of wraps and sweats has been extensively documented. Some tribes even had several different sweat lodges for various purposes—some for relaxation, others for ceremonial use, still others for bathing.

The person who gave me the Pueblo People Wrap was not a Native American, but she certainly embodied the ceremonial spirit of the region. Her name was Susan, and she greeted me near the spa desk with a wide smile. She had short brown hair and sparkling brown eyes.

Leading me back into the treatment room, she had me lie facedown on a massage table prepared with warm muslin sheets. She rubbed a mixture of lavender/sage oil and rosehip/aloe lotion into my skin, covering my legs first and moving up onto my back.

I noticed that each time she finished spreading this mixture on one area, she immediately wrapped that part of my body. This kept me warm and gave me a sense of protection. When she was finished with the back, I turned over, and she repeated the process, from the tips of my toes up to my head, wrapping as she went.

During the twenty minutes that I remained wrapped, Susan massaged my head, face, and hands, and then she moved down to my feet, unwrapping only the area she was working on at the time.

Slowly and softly, as I lay wrapped on the table, Susan's hands and her attention started to work their magic. The first thing I noticed were her fingers getting hotter. They seemed to melt into my skin as she touched me. Then she slowed her movements and her breathing, bringing it into sync with mine. A vibrating energy began to rise in my spine. I felt suddenly like laughing and crying at the same time. And far in the background, quiet and subtle, I thought I heard chanting voices and a drumbeat, like Indian families from long ago doing ceremonies right on this same spot.

I thought I was hallucinating, and I asked Susan what kind of special technique she was using to get her hands so hot and to get my energy so in tune with hers. She looked down at me and smiled. "When people ask what kind of technique I use in the spa services and massage I give," she said, "I tell them it's the *love* technique. I'm tuning in to you and intuitively giving what I feel you need."

With that, she laid one hot hand over my chest. The other she placed on my forehead. The current of pleasure that shot between those two places was unmistakable. She spent another ten minutes massaging my head and neck, leaving me finally in a state of energized bliss.

Then she left me there on the table alone, wrapped from head to foot, like one of the Pueblo people, a person in tune with the forces around him. And the canyon walls spoke to me for days afterward.

In the following sections, I am going to share with you a simple wrapping procedure similar to the one used at Enchantment. You won't need to tune in to the energy of the Pueblo people. Rather, simply listen to your own heart, and do what comes naturally.

The Loving Touch

Susan gives the Pueblo People Wrap at a resort named Enchantment in the middle of a sacred Indian canyon in the red-rock desert. You may live in the suburbs of a midwestern city, but you can still create an experience like the one Susan creates. You can share a tremendous loving energy with those whom you choose to touch. And they will definitely feel the difference.

What is the secret of the loving touch? One word—*attention*. You will have to pay close loving attention to every gesture and intention during your treatment. You'll have to focus on your own inner energy, as you'll learn to do in the next chapter. You will have to drop every other agenda in your life for those few minutes, remembering only to care deeply for the person whom you are touching.

Many spa therapists have a few useful techniques to get themselves prepared for this deep level of giving. You can use them too.

Loving Attention Techniques

1. Before you begin a treatment, rub your hands together vigorously until you feel heat radiating from them. Hold the palms together in stillness for a moment, then place them over your heart, then outward toward your partner.

2. When you are touching someone, close your eyes and imagine that it is your own body you are touching. How would you like to feel? What would you like those hands to do next?

3. Take the time to "listen" for the response that the person's skin and muscles give you when you touch them. Don't just touch and move on. Touch, wait for your partner's response, then respond to her in turn. In that way, touch becomes a dance of two-way communication.

4. Feel for the subtle energies in your partner's body. There are many different systems for coming into tune with these energies, but even without any training at all, you can teach yourself how to pay attention on other levels beyond the physical. One technique is to lift your palms a few inches from your partner's skin and feel for areas of greater and

lesser heat. When you come across a "hot" area, gently place your palm down on the spot. Simply by paying attention in this way, you'll be creating a new kind of awareness within yourself and your partner.

A LOVE WRAP

You Will Need:

- Two tablespoons of aromatherapy massage oil mixed together with half a cup of skin conditioning lotion. Lavender/sage oil is especially nice, and rosehip/aloe lotion is great, but any high-quality ingredients will do. Don't wait until you have the right stuff to begin loving!

- One spa sheet. Muslin is best, but flannel and pure cotton are good too. If the room you're in is cool, place a wool blanket beneath the sheet so you can wrap your partner in that as well.

Step by Step

1. With your partner facedown on the sheet, warm a dab of the oil/lotion mixture between your palms. Begin spreading the mixture onto her skin, starting on one calf and moving up. Finish the first leg, then go on to the next, taking your time, paying attention, feeling for a response, and responding in turn. Give luxury and sensual awareness to your partner. As you finish with each leg, pull the edges of the sheet up to wrap and keep it warm.

2. Continue with the massage, spreading your mixture onto your partner's back.

3. Have your partner turn over, and begin massaging the mixture onto one leg first, then the other, covering each with the sheet as you finish.

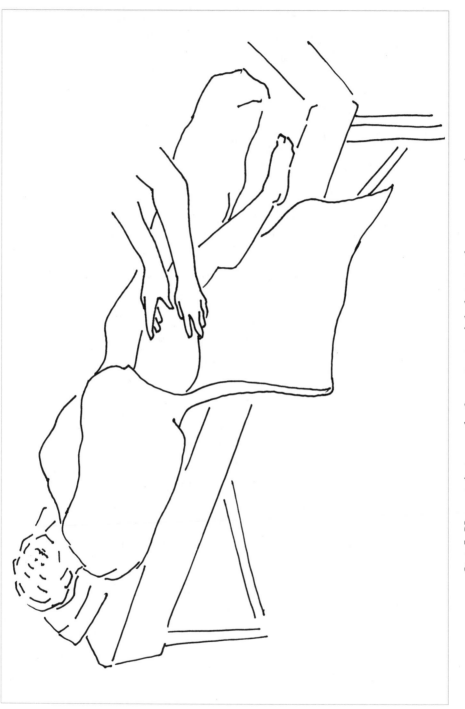

Step 5: Unwrap just enough of your partner's body to touch one area at a time.

4. Spread the lotion onto the torso and arms, then finish the wrap, making sure your partner is comfortable. Does she need a pillow beneath her neck or her knees? Is she thirsty, uncomfortable in any way?

5. While your partner is wrapped for twenty minutes, massage her scalp, neck, and face. Unwrap just enough of the sheet to reach one hand at a time, then one foot at a time. How would you want *your* body to be touched right now? Go slowly, much more slowly than you'd think. Pay attention.

6. You may want to let your partner just drift for a time while she's still wrapped. Often people will automatically go into a meditative state at this point.

7. As you gently unwrap the sheet from around her, run your hands palm-down over your partner's body, a few inches away, just feeling. If an area of particular warmth or intensity stands out, allow your palm to come to rest there. Breathe with her. Communicate without words.

8. To finish, place one palm over her heart and the other over her forehead. Make the connection. Feel the energy. If you're quiet enough and listen closely, you may even hear the subtle echoes of drumbeats in the background.

A Love Wrap is an excellent, simple way to show how much you care for someone. No special expertise is required. However, your partner's experience will be enhanced if you practice the massage techniques from the previous chapter.

"People are coming here [to my new Center for Well Being], I think, for one thing, whether or not they have a disease—for improving the quality of their life, not just when they're here, but when they go home."

—Dr. Deepak Chopra

✾ *Chapter 10* ✾

THE PLEASURES OF AYURVEDA

Chopra Center for Well Being, La Jolla, California

The rocky coast along La Jolla in southern California rises up from cold Pacific waves, where seals sun themselves and surfers plunge forever back toward the land. Hot air balloons hang as if motionless in the clear sky, floating gumdrops. And all along the grassy parks and the patches of sand at the city's edge, people gather for picnics on weekend afternoons, looking around at the surrounding scene every few minutes as if to remind themselves that it is real.

A few blocks inland, on a quiet street where the ocean can no longer be seen but where it can still be felt and heard, I found a newly refurbished building with a burnished metal plaque fastened near the door—The Chopra Center for Well Being.

The center had opened its doors only two weeks earlier. The ocher paint on the outer walls was still fresh, making the large two-story building glow in the afternoon light. It has a solid churchlike grandeur, with arches and graceful curves, and perhaps it is a kind of church, although most people know it simply as the newest and most innovative mind-body "spa" in the country. Dr. Deepak Chopra, famous for his many books on healing and spirituality, created the center to be the heart of his life's work, and people from all over the world have already set their sights on visiting it. The basic philosophy and lifestyle taught here are founded on the ancient principles of Ayurveda, a five-thousand-year-old system of health and healing from India.

Stepping through the front door and past the earthy stone-paved lobby, I found myself in the Store of Infinite Possibilities. This shop was filled with hundreds of the latest volumes about health, healing, massage, nutrition, and consciousness. I wanted to stay all day, to pore through several books while sipping herbal tea and savoring a delight or two in the all-natural café, Quantum Soup.

But other delights were awaiting me.

A young woman named Jennifer led me down a hallway past conference rooms that were named after the seven spiritual laws. Meditation classes, yoga therapy, and private consultations are given in these rooms throughout the day. Farther on, we entered the treatment room area. The rooms here are named for various principles as well—Karma, Giving, Potentiality, and what was to be my own treatment room, Least Effort.

After Jennifer had me sit down, she placed a small curved pillow over the back of my neck. It was filled with seeds that had been heated to just the right temperature, and the sensation of toasty warmth immediately began to sink into my muscles. Then just before she left, Jennifer reached out her hand and touched me on the shoulder for a couple of seconds. "Your therapists will be here in just a moment," she said. "Have a wonderful treatment." She smiled as she turned away, and I thought about how special that was, to be touched by someone when it wasn't part of the treatment. Just that extra bit of human warmth started the flow of healing energy in my system.

A moment later *two* therapists, Colleen and Clinton, entered the room and explained what I was about to experience. The Odyssey treatment is a blending of several of the best therapies at the Chopra Center. When I signed up for it, I knew I was in for a treat, but I had no idea that both a man and a woman would be working on me at the same time.

Both Colleen and Clinton were thin and graceful. In fact, it turned out that Colleen had studied dance for quite a while. They had that particular glow to the skin and the clarity of the eyes that betokens a healthful vegetarian lifestyle. As I lay down on my back on the treatment table in the room of Least Effort, they explained to me that the Odyssey would be administered in silence. All three of us allowed our minds as well as our mouths to become still.

Each donning a pair of natural-fiber gloves, Colleen and Clinton stood on either side of the table, took a deep breath in unison with each other and with me, then began.

Immediately I was transported. Their every movement was choreographed and precise, and yet there was a spontaneity and freedom to them as well. Four hands raced over my skin, with the roughly textured gloves sloughing off dead cells and accumulated karma, it seemed, at the same time. This part of the Odyssey is called *Garshana* in the Ayurvedic tradition, a type of exfoliation (see Chapter 3). It lasted for a good fifteen minutes, until my skin tingled and glowed. I was instructed to turn over, and the process was repeated with exquisite precision on the part of both therapists.

After this cleansing, they both poured generous amounts of a warmed sesame, sunflower, and safflower oil blend into their palms and began a massage. Their synchronized movements started out slow and then increased in speed and depth. This part of the treatment is known as *Vishesh,* and it is meant to loosen impurities and relieve tension on a deep level. Colleen worked on my feet while Clinton massaged my head. Then I became lost, unable to keep track of whose hands were where, as seemingly by magic both of my hands, my feet, and my heart were being touched at the same time. A great pleasure-bringing Being took me over, a four-handed Power that had me in its grip. The massage finally became light again toward the end, touching just upon the most sensitive energized points.

This was definitely a time for practicing Conscious Pleasure Principle Number 6—Surrender to Pleasure. When two people are doing their best to bring you bodily bliss and healing, it's easy to flip over into a puritanical inability to receive. Each time a thought like that occurred, I reminded myself of the sixth principle once again, until the nagging voice of self-denial finally quieted down.

When it was over an hour later, a few moments of total silence and stillness ensued. Then suddenly something moist and very warm was spread over my body, first in one spot, then all over, and I relaxed even further as several large hot towels were plied into my skin.

Moments later, just as my skin began to cool, warm blankets were wrapped around me, and I was told to slide toward the head of the table. My head was placed back in a sling, and Colleen draped a towel over my eyes. Then she released a tiny stream of warmed oil directly onto my forehead. This is known as *Shirod-hara;* the stream of oil was pouring over my "third eye," which is supposed to effect the integration of body and mind.

Silently I waited for a connection between body and soul. What I felt instead was something unexpected and deeply luxurious. The steady stream of oil started on my forehead first, then slowly pooled up into my hairline, then back through my hair to the top of my head, and finally all the way back over my scalp. A warm, slow-moving river washed over my whole head, with the extra oil dripping down through the sling into a receptacle below.

After what seemed like a gallon of the warmed oil had slalomed through my now slick and nourished hair, Colleen stopped the flow. She then ran her fingers over my head, massaging my scalp, face, and neck for a few last moments while Clinton slipped out of the room.

"Wow," I said at last, my first word for almost two hours. "That was incredible."

"Isn't it wonderful?" said Colleen. "The science of Ayurveda has used a natural system of therapies called *panchakarma* for five thousand years. You just received a sampling of several of them. People on a *panchakarma* program receive massage and other treatments every day and eat a specified diet as well. Meditation is also a big part of it. It's a way of life that helps bring people back into a healthy balance with themselves and their environment. Many people have healed serious illnesses by following this system."

Colleen helped me sit up and then slipped sticky little slippers onto my feet so I wouldn't slide on the tile floor when I stood up. So much oil is used during the treatments that this has become a necessary precaution.

After a hot shower I wandered upstairs to the dining room to have lunch with the staff and guests. All of them were happy to share their knowledge. Ayurvedic therapies, they told me, treat a person's *prakruti,* or basic nature. And that nature is in turn a combination of different mind-body types, or *doshas.* Two medical doctors help guests gain an understanding of their condition and how Ayurveda might benefit them. A knowledgeable staff of nutritionists, herbalists, counselors, yoga teachers, chefs, coordinators, therapists, and assistants all work together to make this new center something more than a typical spa.

Of course, Deepak Chopra is the inspiration behind the operation. Through his books and speaking engagements, he spreads interest about natural healing, higher consciousness, and spirituality everywhere he goes. His office is down the hall from the dining room. When I spoke with him, I asked how his new center will fit into the mainstream of the spa world.

"I think the spa philosophy is still in evolution," he said in his melodic East Indian accent. "It very much has been body-based, and what we need to do now is get several levels further, so that when a person comes to a healing center such as ours, my hope is that everything is addressed: their physical body, their emotional subtle body, their intellectual body, and their spiritual body. And therefore, along with the massage and the bodily based treatments, they should always be in an educational process. There should be some component that gives spiritual experience in the form of meditation. And there should be a dynamic that nourishes release in the emotional body.

"I think healing is much more than getting rid of a disease or pain. People are coming here, I think, for one thing, whether or not they have a disease—for improving the quality of their life, not just when they're here but when they go home."

HOME JOURNEY

You can create a treatment similar to the Odyssey on your own at home. Remember, the word *odyssey* means "journey," and the pleasure you experience in giving or receiving this treatment will not depend on whether you do it "right." You probably have not undergone months of Ayurvedic training or spent countless hours perfecting your massage choreography, but that doesn't matter. What matters is entering into a journey, going through it, and coming out on the other end refreshed, revitalized, and centered. Here is a treatment I recommend for a journey to revitalization.

For Yourself

Preparation

Make sure you have two hand towels in your STU, ready to go. You'll also need a loofah sponge or mitt and a bottle of massage oil.

Step by Step

1. First, seated in a comfortable chair with a towel beneath you, slough off your dead skin with the loofah, taking special care to use thorough circular movements around the elbows, heels, and any rough areas. Depending on the type of loofah, you can either use it dry or moisten it slightly for comfort. Cover as much of your skin as you can reach, and make the process vigorous! This is not just for exfoliation but to get the circulation and lymphatic drainage going as well. Aim long strokes with the loofah back toward the heart.

2. Pour a liberal amount of massage oil into your palm, and give yourself a massage, working first on your calves, knees, and thighs, then working up to your abdomen. Rub warmed oil into your tummy, slowly and languorously. Let the indulgence be complete as you enjoy the feel of yourself. Run your palms up over your chest and onto your shoulders. One hand glides toward the other and massages it for a minute. Then they switch roles. Allow both hands to reach up behind your neck, kneading there, then finish with your face and scalp (see Self-Massage in Chapter 8).

3. This time, as you reverse the direction and massage your way back down your body, be more aggressive, working knots and tension as you descend from head to neck to arms to torso to legs. Finish by gently placing your palms over any areas that feel the need for love or special attention. Concentrate on the area, sending acceptance and healing energy.

4. Reach into the STU and withdraw the first of your towels. Open it, and wrap the hot cloth around one leg, sliding it up, then the other leg. Open the next hot towel and place it directly upon your belly. Then move it up over your shoulders, arms, and hands.

5. When you feel smooth and clean, lie back down into your comfy chair, or recline upon the bed or floor. Pull the edges of a blanket up over your body and get snuggled in.

6. Dribble a few drops of oil on the tip of your middle finger, and then rub that finger in tiny circles around the area in the center of your forehead, above the bridge of the nose, known as the "third eye." Massage there for a few minutes, breathing in and out slowly and focusing on the sense of openness and inner awareness this brings. This spot stimulates the pineal gland, which regulates the function of other glands. This in turn benefits the entire hormonal system of the body.

7. Lie still for several minutes when you have finished, soaking up the relaxation and basking in a new awareness.

For Your Partner

You Will Need:

Two hot hand towels in the STU

A loofah mitt or sponge

Massage oil

Step by Step

1. With you partner lying on his back, begin with a quick brushing of the skin with your sponge or mitt. Make sure the surface has a little texture to it but is not too rough. The direction of the brushing is generally toward the heart. Use circles around the navel.

2. Turn your partner onto his stomach, and continue the brushing for a few more minutes.

3. Pour a liberal amount of warmed massage oil into one palm, rub your hands together, and begin with an easy, long-stroke-style massage (see Chapter 8) that gradually becomes a little firmer.

4. Have your partner turn over, and repeat the massage strokes on the front of the body.

5. When you are finished with the massage, just gently touch your partner on the points where you intuitively feel he needs soothing. Hold your palms there for a minute at a time, not moving or doing, just concentrating on radiating positive healing energy.

6. Pull the edges of a blanket or spa sheet up around your partner to keep him warm and make him feel protected.

7. Using only an ounce of warmed massage oil, pour it as slowly as possible in a steady stream down over your partner's forehead, directly over the "third eye." This is a good time to suggest some positive visualizations or affirmations, if you think

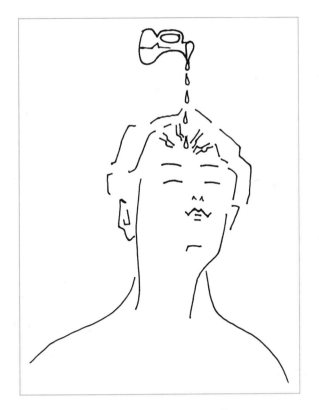

Step 7: Pour a warm stream of oil over your partner's "third eye."

it's appropriate. Make sure his head is tilted back and that he has a towel underneath.

8. Do a slow deep scalp massage, luxuriously working the oil into his hair and skin.

Note: For an added touch of luxury, try another technique similar to that used at the Chopra Center. Just before you start your Journey treatment, place a warmed neck pillow over your shoulders and around the back of your neck. The same ones used at the Chopra Center are listed in Appendix A. If you don't have a professional pillow, just take a hand towel straight from the clothes dryer, roll it up, and wrap it over yourself like a stole. The warmth will remain for five or ten minutes.

THE DOUBLE TOUCH

The experience I had in the room of Least Effort was extra special because two therapists were working on me at the same time. And the effect was exponential: it was more than the pleasure of a normal massage and more than that pleasure doubled. It was massage squared. Massage to the second power.

If you've never experienced it before, this is something you should definitely create for yourself. And you don't need two friends who have an expert choreographed routine to offer. One night before bedtime, offer your foot up to be squeezed by your husband and one hand to be stroked by a daughter or son. You will be absolutely amazed. In our society there is something of an unspoken taboo about group touching of any kind. If you break through this taboo, consciously and with love, what you'll find on the other side is practically an overload of healthy, pleasurable sensations. Two bodies, two loving hearts, four tender hands touching you with attention and care, feel like an entire legion of beings devoted to your every need. There is something ultimately indulgent

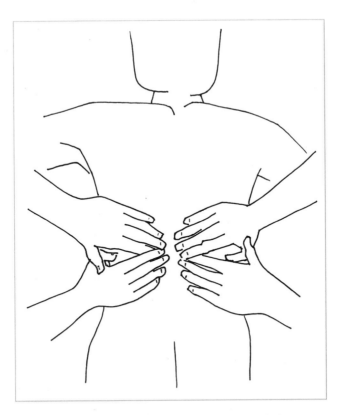

Four hands touching you is the ultimate indulgence.

and royal about it. Try this quick fifteen-minute experience, and I'm sure you'll feel like Cleopatra before it's over.

Step by Step

1. You lie on the floor, thoroughly cushioned with pillows and blankets. There's no need to disrobe for this one; just wear loose comfortable clothing.

2. Your two partners start at either side of your chest, kneeling or sitting. Simultaneously they lay their hands upon your heart and your belly, holding them there for a minute. Feel the full power of those four hands holding you spread through every cell. At this point, it's very hard not to surrender. So go ahead and do it. Take a deep breath. Let go.

3. Each partner takes a hand and begins a slow, careful five-minute massage of your fingers, palm, wrist, and forearm. For details on hand massage, see page 90.

4. One partner slides quietly down to your feet while the other pivots to sit above your head. For the next seven or eight minutes you'll be receiving a foot massage and a head/neck/shoulder massage simultaneously, which is just about the closest thing to heaven this side of childhood. For details on these massage techniques, see pages 88 and 91.

5. Finish with the partners coming back to your sides again, gently settling their palms over your heart and belly. Open your eyes, and look up into theirs. Chances are you'll be feeling more than just ultra-relaxed; a tear or two might form in the corner of your eye. Being cared for on this level often brings with it an emotional fulfillment so deep that you suddenly realize it was something you were desperately yearning for all along, although you didn't know it.

MEDITATION

As Dr. Chopra has made so clear, it is not really the massage or the oil or the heated towel or even the contact with another person that is at the root of healing or consciousness pleasure. He says that the most important facet of a full mind-body spa experience is "the experience of meditation and transcending, experiencing your soul and spirit."

Meditation, in fact, usually is a part of any great spa treatment. A certain silent synchronicity happens between therapist and client, and often between the client and her Self. In this space of togetherness and unity, the constant chatter of the internal voice shuts itself off for a time. It is from this realm of inner quiet that deep healing emerges.

The following is a five-minute meditation exercise that you can use separately or during any of the spa treatments in this book.

Step by Step

1. Sit comfortably, either on a chair or upon a cushion on the floor. Make sure your back is properly supported and your spine is straight. Your legs can be either folded or extended, and your arms positioned so that your hands rest lightly on your thighs, palms facing upward.

2. Closing your eyes, take a deep, deep breath, much deeper than you think you need to take, so deep that you cannot possibly pull any more oxygen into your lungs. Exhale. Repeat the breath, this time even deeper.

3. Let your breathing normalize. Then, keeping conscious track of your breathing, begin gradually to let every other thought that enters your head slip right back out again. Concentrate on only one thing—your breath.

4. As your thoughts begin to slow down, allow space for new awareness to filter in. Each time you inhale or exhale fully without getting caught in a new thought, you will sink further into connection with your body, that old friend that most of the time is just along for the ride we take it on with our minds. For these moments, let your body *be* your mind. "Think" with your body, and feel with your body too.

5. Each time a thought comes, go back to your breath. Just be.

6. If you feel the urge to let a sound or a movement escape you, go for it! A loud "Praise me!" is appropriate, or just a whoop of inchoate joy. This is the sound of your inner Self expressing itself. Movements might include a stretch, an energetic yawn, or rapid in-and-out breathing. Allow energy to circulate through you.

7. A time will naturally come when you feel like opening your eyes. (It could be after five minutes, it could be after an hour.) Obey your natural urge, and come back gradually.

8. Thank yourself for this, the most valuable time you can spend. Know that coming more fully into contact with your own

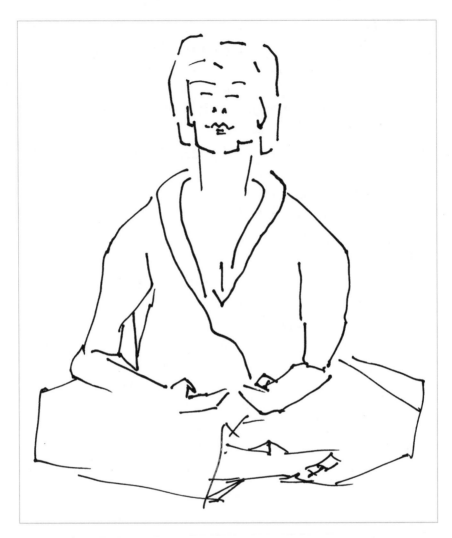

Step 5: Just be.

mind-body is the most direct route to fulfilling your highest aspirations.

If you want a direct connection to the Store of Infinite Possibilities at the Chopra Center, call (619) 551-7130. The experts on herbs and other natural healing products who work there can give you recommendations.

For further information about Ayurveda and body treatments:

Chopra, Dr. Deepak. *Return of the Rishi*. New York: Houghton Mifflin, 1988.

Chopra, Dr. Deepak. *Unconditional Life*. New York: Bantam Books, 1991.

Johari, Harish. *Ayurvedic Massage*. Rochester, Vt.: Healing Arts Press, 1996.

Lad, Dr. Vasant. *Ayurveda, The Science of Self-Healing*. Santa Fe: Lotus Press, 1984.

Sachs, Melanie. *Ayurvedic Beauty Care*. Twin Lakes, Wisc.: Lotus Press, 1994.

*"To me, the sea is like a person—like a child that
I've known for a long time. When I swim in the sea
I talk to it. I never feel alone when I'm out there."*
—Gertrude Ederle
first woman to swim the English Channel

❦ *Chapter 11* ❧

KELP HELPS—SPA TREATMENTS WITH SEAWEED

Canyon Ranch in the Berkshires, Lenox, Massachusetts

In the Berkshire Mountains of Massachusetts, locked in on every side by land as far as the eye can see, a spa retreat exists where the powerful healing energy of the sea is harnessed every day, even though the sea itself is hundreds of miles away. The name of the spa is Canyon Ranch, and it enjoys one of the loftiest reputations of all the great spa resorts. The original Canyon Ranch is in Tucson, Arizona, and for many years people have made the pilgrimage out to the desert for some serious concentration on health and fitness. The sister property in the Northeast is newer, but it enjoys an equally high reputation.

The spa is built around the Bellefontaine Mansion, a grand old estate that in turn is patterned after one of the buildings at Ver-

The Royal Treatment

133

sailles in France. Sleek new glass wings have been added to the original turn-of-the-century structure, and the entire complex is connected so that nobody has to leave the building in case of inclement weather.

I arrived in November, and several inches of crisp snow already lay over the grounds. Cold hills surrounded the resort, and the stark bare branches of trees made whistling noises as the New England wind swept through them. Inside, though, I knew that a warm inviting chamber was being prepared for me. I was scheduled to receive a seaweed body treatment.

Once inside the resort's inviting doors, I was struck by how extensive the facilities are. Multiple gymnasiums, pools, indoor tennis courts, and conference rooms sprawl throughout the multilayered complex. Separate men's and women's wet areas branch off near a sparkling clean spa reception desk.

Tonya Defriest, my therapist, greeted me in the lobby and led me down a hallway to the seaweed room. She is a slender, aristocratic-looking young woman with straight blond hair. The walls inside her treatment room were green like seaweed, and the rich organic smell of the seashore hit my nostrils as soon as I entered. I was reminded of the time I'd spent at the Ihilani spa in Hawaii. The therapeutic powers of the sea were only a few hundred feet from the spa's wet area there. Now here I was in New England. Snow lay on the ground outside, and the warm waters of that lagoon in the Pacific were half a world away. Yet the main ingredient of a true sea-healing was right there in the room with me—*Digita laminaria,* better known as seaweed.

In this case, the seaweed was reconstituted from sea plants harvested from the waters off the northwestern shores of Normandy, in France. The spa industry is a major consumer of the world's supply of therapeutic algaes, and most of it comes from this part of the globe. Boats head out to the vast kelp beds far offshore, bringing back thick tangles of the mineral-rich plants. These are then processed at factories, where they are transformed into the powders and pastes used in spas. Several health spas that specialize in sea treatments can be found right there on the shores of France where the products are made. These are known as *balneotherapy* centers, the root *balneo* meaning "bath."

More than eight hundred types of seaweed can be found in the world. Dozens of them are eaten by many cultures, but only seven or eight are used for cosmetic and healing purposes. Of these few, kelp is the most popular, with white and brown algae close behind. Reconstituted spa algaes are usually a mixture of kelp and one other type of seaweed.

During my spa training workshops, I explain to students how similar our blood is to seawater. The molecules are nearly the same, and in fact when there is a shortage of plasma during wartime, seawater is often substituted. The secret to sea treatments is in this similarity. During a Seaweed Wrap our bodies soak in the vast store of nutrients and minerals found in seawater and plants right through the skin, as if we were receiving a transfusion!

Once several years ago I had an opportunity to witness the amazing properties of seaweed while working at another New England spa resort, called Topnotch in Stowe, Vermont, where I was in charge of hiring and training a staff of therapists. Since this spa is even farther away from the ocean than the Canyon Ranch, several of the therapists were not familiar with seaweed treatments, and many of the guests who came to the spa in the beginning were a little skeptical as well.

Carole Spellman, the spa director at Topnotch at the time, realized that this was not unusual. "If you're not from Europe or California," she commented, "chances are you may not understand the benefits of seaweed treatments. This is changing more every day, but education will always play an important role in helping guests get the most out of their treatments."

It is not necessary to know every nutrient found in seaweed in order to benefit from a Seaweed Wrap, but the list is quite impressive, and seeing it will give you an idea of the complexity and depth of this natural product. Whenever you apply organic seaweeds to your skin, you will be soaking in through your pores a combination of nitrogen, phosphorous, potassium, sulfur, magnesium, calcium, iodine, iron, manganese, cobalt, copper, zinc, bromine, amino acids, vitamins, phytohormones, and antibacterial agents. Many seaweed products also contain some essential oils, such as cinnamon, rosemary, sage, peppermint, eucalyptus, pine, juniper, lavender, and others. With this combination of powerful ingredients, you are sure to derive multiple benefits from any treatment involving seaweed. And there is no need to worry about which particular products are recommended for each person. Seaweed treatments are good for all skin types, especially for dry and sun-damaged skin.

While training at the spa at Topnotch, we hired an expert in French seaweeds, Annette Hanson, to come up and give us further information. She instructed us in the three R's of seaweed treatments:

1. Remineralization
2. Revitalization
3. Rejuvenation

The primary benefit is Remineralization. Because of the depletion of our soil, air, and water, the crops that we grow today do not have the same vitamin and mineral content that they did in the days of our grandparents and great-grandparents. What we eat, breathe, and drink are devitalized versions of the original elements. For this reason it is especially important to find some auxiliary way to replenish our bodies. Seaweed is one of the best ways available. As it soaks through our skin during a wrap, we absorb an almost perfect source of nutrition into our cells, especially when the seaweed has been harvested from areas like Normandy, where pollution levels are very low.

Back in the treatment room at Canyon Ranch, Tonya began the procedure by having me lie between two warmed sheets. She proceeded to cleanse my skin with a loose-woven loofah and a gentle exfoliant. After this was repeated on both sides of my body, she had me step into a shower that was conveniently just inches away.

This room had been designed specifically with seaweed treatments in mind, and the shower was an integral part of it.

The sheets were changed, and an extra layer was added on the bottom—plastic this time. I slipped between them face-up, and Tonya used the light touch of her thin, graceful hands to apply a warmed mixture of seaweed and essential oils. When my body was covered, Tonya wrapped me in the layer of plastic first, and then a sheet and blanket. I could already feel the minerals starting to soak into my body. My body heat was being reflected back from the plastic sheet, helping the absorption process.

"Would you like me to leave the lights on low or turn them off altogether?" asked Tonya, her voice feather-soft so as not to disturb my impending trance.

"I think I'd like them turned off," I told her.

Tonya is an excellent therapist who started at the spa a few years ago in the hospitality department as a guest services specialist. "I had a feeling I'd enjoy doing treatments," she told me, "and so I signed up for school and kept working here at Canyon Ranch while learning the techniques. Now I couldn't imagine doing anything else. This is definitely the highest level of giving and serving that I've ever experienced. I think it'll be a lifelong career for me."

She turned off the lights and quietly shut the door behind her. I was left in the warm darkened room with gentle music floating down from the ceiling somewhere, and before I slipped into the nowhere-land between sleeping and meditation, I thought about what Tonya had said. It's true; people who choose to work in the spa world are the most giving people around. Either consciously or unconsciously, they choose to spend many hours of every day making other people feel whole, healthy, and alive. What better course to choose?

Then, for the next twenty minutes, I indulged myself in Conscious Pleasure Principle Number 6—Surrender to Pleasure. When Tonya came back in the room, I was in an altered state, and she brought the lights up very gradually to ease me out of it.

"How was that?" she asked.

"Out of this world."

"I know. Seaweed Wraps are the best. My only problem is that I don't get one often enough. I try wrapping myself, but the logistics just don't work."

Once again she helped me up and into the shower. While I scrubbed off seaweed, she prepared the table one last time. Then I lay between new sheets, and she applied some emollient lotion that had seaweed extracts in it. While she massaged it in, she smiled at me bashfully and said, "I have a confession to make. This is the first time I've given a Seaweed Wrap to a man. I didn't know how I was going to arrange the sheets and towels to make you comfortable while doing a thorough treatment, but I hope it was good enough, because we're getting a lot more requests from men for this type of procedure."

"You seemed like an old pro to me," I told her. "Everything was as smooth as could be. If you hadn't mentioned it, I never would have known."

THE SEAWEED WRAP

Preparation

You are going to create a simplified version of the Seaweed Wrap in your own home. The following technique follows the format I teach to my students in spa workshops, except for one particular detail. In the workshops no showers are available, and so each student has the opportunity to experience seaweed being peeled from their body with a spatula and hot towels! A shower is preferable. Set up your Seaweed Wrap as close to the shower as possible. This will make it easier for your partner and also keep her warmer.

If you are going to use preblended seaweed, simply warm it up. An electric warmer or double boiler is better than a microwave for this purpose. If you choose to mix your own from powdered seaweed and essential oils, follow the directions that come with the powder, adding enough water to create a batterlike consistency. After being reconstituted, seaweed can last up to two weeks in the refrigerator. Just make sure to warm it up when you're about to start the treatment.

In successive layers place a blanket, a sheet, and a piece of plastic (such as a split-open plastic trash bag) down on the carpeting or on a massage table. In many spas a metallic fabric known as Mylar is used instead of plastic to reflect the person's heat back into the wrap. This substance is very expensive, however, and it carries the added disadvantage of being very bad for the environment. In my spa workshops I switched to biodegradable plastic because this part of the wrap is going to be discarded. You can use an old sheet instead, but it will not retain body heat well, and it will become messy.

A word of caution: This wrap is not recommended for people who are allergic to shellfish. That allergy is most often caused by a reaction to iodine, which is present in seaweed. Wrapping oneself up in the very substance one is allergic to can lead to some itchy situations. Actually, among the hundreds of people I've wrapped in spas and in spa workshops, only one had any reaction to the seaweed, but it is always much better to be safe than sorry. Therefore, if you or your partner is allergic to shellfish, you might want to forgo a seaweed treatment.

You Will Need:

- A loofah sponge
- A small amount of exfoliant
- For wrapping: a blanket, a sheet, a plastic sheet
- Body lotion
- 4 ounces of prepared seaweed

You can buy seaweed body masque in beauty supply stores and some department stores. A good source is also listed in Appendix A.

Step by Step

1. Have your partner lie down on the table face-up. Drape her with a towel or sheet, making sure to keep her warm.

2. Using a soft dry loofah, gently rub away any traces of dead skin cells, excess oil, or dirt that may hinder the penetration of the seaweed into the pores.

3. Have your partner turn over, and repeat the exfoliation on the back.

4. Begin applying seaweed in long slow movements, using your hands or a natural-bristle paintbrush and covering each area of the body with the wrap as soon as you're finished in order to keep your partner warm.

5. Have her turn over, and finish the application on the front. Seaweed can be applied to the breasts (that's the way they do it in France), but be careful about applications to the face. The skin there may be too delicate. There are special seaweeds produced especially for that purpose.

6. Completely wrap your partner with the plastic secured around her body and tucked all around with the sheet and blanket. Place a pillow under her knees to support the lower back.

7. Now you can leave her alone for twenty minutes, with the lights turned down low and soft music playing. Or if she prefers, apply a seaweed face mask (see page 143).

8. After twenty minutes, unwrap your partner. Make sure that the hot water in the shower is already turned on because it is *guaranteed* that she will be cold when she comes out of the nice warm wrap.

9. While she showers, dispose of the plastic and lay out a clean towel or sheet.

10. Have her lie down again after she's dried off. Apply some moisturizing body lotion in a quick five-minute routine, or if you're feeling generous, make this the beginning of a full-

body Spa Massage. Make sure to use lotion instead of oil for the entire massage, to replenish moisture in the pores.

SEAWEED SELF-WRAP

As Tonya pointed out, it is difficult to give a Seaweed Wrap to yourself. But a friend in the spa industry has tipped me off about a very decent wrap that you can do yourself in the bathtub. The simple procedure is as follows.

Step by Step

1. In a dry bathtub, stretch out a wool blanket, a sheet, and a piece of plastic.

2. Run a soft loofah over your skin for two minutes to exfoliate.

3. Sit down in the tub on top of the plastic, and apply four ounces of warmed seaweed all over your body, from your toes upward.

4. Pull the layers of wrapping around you and lie back in the tub. With a little foresight, you'll remember to have a pillow ready behind your head.

5. Stay wrapped for fifteen to twenty minutes, with a candle glowing in the room and soft music playing. You'll be surprised how comfortable you can get, wrapped up snug in a bathtub.

6. Unwrap yourself, slip the blanket and sheets out of the tub, and immediately begin filling it with warm water. As the seaweed on your skin begins to dissolve in the water, it will create an impromptu seaweed bath, the subject of our next treatment.

7. Finish by drying off and applying some moisturizing lotion to your skin.

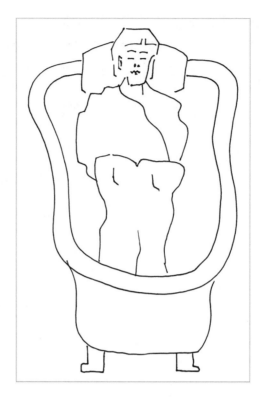

Step 5: You'll be surprised how comfortable you can get.

SEAWEED BATH

Limu is the name they give to seaweed in the Hawaiian Islands, where they use it for its healing properties. In Jamaica they make a special drink from seaweed called Irish moss, which is supposed to cure everything from impotence to anemia. The Japanese are famous for their creative use of seaweeds in the culinary arts. And in America many people eat a species of blue-green algae for increased physical stamina and mental clarity.

Seaweed is good for you. The simplest way you can take advantage of its benefits is to pour some seaweed powder into a bath and soak. (Hydrotherapy Baths are described in Chapter 4.) Plenty of products come prepackaged with the correct amount already selected. For bulk seaweeds, approximately one-quarter cup of powder per tub is plenty. Prepared seaweed pastes are usually a little more difficult to blend into baths; if you try them, mix a quarter cup in one quart of water in a blender first, then add to the bath.

Step by Step

1. Run a warm bath, and while it's filling, use a loofah on your skin for a light exfoliation.
2. When the tub is almost full, add the seaweed.
3. Immerse and enjoy.

Note: Seaweeds are fun to use in Jacuzzis, but be careful about plumbing and jets. Seaweed can cake and dry in the delicate fixtures, creating problems. Also, some algaes tend to foam when subjected to bubbles, and you many end up with a frothy green mess in the bathroom. This happened to me once when I was testing some new products.

SEAWEED FACE MASK

In Chapter 6 we explored a facial treatment (Gentleman's Facial) in which one of the options was a seaweed mask. The mask is easy to apply. Just make sure to get the right products. Certain seaweeds are formulated to congeal on the face, making an easily removable layer.

The mask can be applied:

• During the Seaweed Wrap
• As part of the facial treatment
• Separately on its own, after a long day, to help rejuvenate the skin

Step by Step

1. Cleanse the face with a toner or cosmetic soap.
2. Apply the mask, and leave it on the face for twenty minutes. Usually the seaweed will harden gradually over time.
3. Peel the mask away gently and discard.
4. Apply a nutrient-rich moisturizing lotion, using upward strokes of the fingers.

Caution: Once again, you should be aware that only certain seaweeds have been formulated for use on the face. If you were to use body-wrap seaweed for a face treatment, it might overstimulate the delicate skin in that area. Read labels carefully. Rely on professionals at retail outlets, or purchase from a reputable source.

The sea will always draw us, pulling at our psyches as if its tides were inside our own bodies. It does not matter how far away from the shore we are—still the huge ocean-swollen belly of our planet calls out in water whispers, and we listen. Spa treatments are an excellent way to connect to the ocean once again. Let yourself be drawn into the therapeutic world of seaweed treatments. They are much easier than you might think, and once you've been wrapped up in green, you'll find it to be quite fun!

> *"People get real comfortable with their*
> *features. Nobody gets comfortable with their*
> *hair. Hair trauma. It's the universal thing."*
> —Jamie Lee Curtis

❧ *Chapter 12* ❧

TREATED FROM TOP TO TOE

Green Valley Spa, Saint George, Utah

———

I n *southwestern Utah's spectacular desert,* shimmering on a ridge not far from the fantastic rock formations of Zion and Bryson, is a spa retreat called the Green Valley.

Imagine rocky desert plateaus and towering white limestone mountains. As I hike through this landscape with a small group of new friends, we see the tracks a fox left the night before in the soft red sand. Some of us have decided to attempt rock climbing, scaling beginner cliffs strapped into harness and rope. The sun, at nine-thirty A.M., is already noonday hot. Thousand-year-old Anasazi Indian petroglyphs are etched into the burning rocks all around as we explore narrow canyons and jumbled piles of stratified rock.

My body, in spite of the conditions, is unbelievably light, buoyant even. My muscles feel strong after a week of hiking, and my mind is clear after a series of first-rate treatments given by the staff in the spa, which we can see up on a ridge many miles in the distance now.

The environment, however, does take its toll. Although everything else feels fine, my poor feet are crying out for some attention.

Most of the others in the group echo this concern, slipping their hiking boots off and kneading sore spots whenever the hike master gives us a moment to rest. And our hair, in spite of hats, has been scorched and dried by the sun. What we need is a little royal treatment designed especially for the very top and the very bottom of the body. Everything in between has been wrapped and scrubbed and massaged to no end. How about those soles and our weather-worn hair?

Luckily, Green Valley can come through. Back at the oasis on the hill after our hike, I ask for treatments that address these problem areas, and I am sent to the appropriate experts.

Entering the treatment area at Green Valley is like entering another world. The harsh outer reality of rock and wind is left behind. After I checked in at the spa desk, I was led by a young woman into the inner sanctum. Immediately my senses were engaged by a detailed attention to color. Each day at the Green Valley Spa is devoted to a different color—the energies of that color, its emanations, the feeling that people get when they are surrounded by it. On this day, after yet another rough hike, I was treated to green. Soothing, cooling green. Green was everywhere. A large silver punch bowl was filled with water permeated with the essence of lime. Green floral arrangements adorned the waiting area. In the dining room that day, centerpieces wrought from evergreen branches arched up high between the courses, dwarfing the diners there, humbling us with green.

On other days we'd been treated to yellow and orange and red. Each color of the spectrum had been carefully chosen by spa owner Carole Coombs to reflect the intention of that particular day. After a very short period of time there, your body falls into sync with the natural progression of the spectrum, following a rainbow pattern that begins to feel completely natural. (See the section called "Add Color to Your Days," at the end of this chapter.)

I was led down a green-lit hallway past idyllic murals of celestial scenes. The sounds of murmuring water filled the space as we passed by the Egyptian Room and the Rose Room and several others. A young woman spread cleansing pastes on washcloths and turned the stream of hot water on for me. Towels were hung close by. A bathrobe was prepared, and I slipped into it. Surrounded by such opulence, I could not help but appreciate Conscious Pleasure Principle Number 2—Ambience.

Next, I was led through another doorway to receive the Hot Oil Pack Hair Treatment. When I glanced up, long willow branches were swaying in a soft desert breeze, and a wind chime played in the slender green leaves. We were outside but in a completely secluded garden. The therapist, Kim, was waiting there with a warm greeting. As I sat in a comfortable chair, she rubbed some natural botanical desert compounds into my hair. The special ingredients had been blended right there at the spa in a laboratory down the hall from the treatment rooms. Essential oil of peppermint tingled my scalp.

After this preparatory stage Kim took a whipped mixture of honey, essential oils, coconut oil, soybean oil, olive oil, and jojoba oil and massaged it into my hair for twenty minutes. Then she instructed me to lie upon a nearby massage table. Once I was lying down, she wrapped my head in four hot towels.

As I lay there, the ravages of the surrounding desert forgotten now, Kim massaged my chest, arms, hands, and feet for another twenty minutes while a superfine mist of cooled water rained down over my body from miniature sprinklers hidden in the willow. Then, surprisingly, she shampooed my hair while I was still lying down, pouring a pitcher of cool purified water over my head and letting the excess run down off the table. She lathered in natural soaps and conditioners for several more minutes, sat me back in the chair to towel me dry, and then sent me back into the cool green maze of the spa's treatment chambers.

Care of the Hair

Cristin Coombs works in the spa's laboratory putting together ingredients like mineral salts, citric extract, crushed pearls, yucca root, coconut, flower blossoms, amber, myrrh, ginger and juniper berries, cinnamon, aloe, sage, rainwater, and potato. These form the compounds used in treatments at the spa, and each compound has a name: Ashes, Sand, Breeze, Honey Dew, Clarity, and Radiance. Cristin takes pride in her work, and the end results are some beautiful products that are great to use at home as well as at the spa. But when you are preparing your own home spa treatments, you needn't feel that you have to be as thorough as they are at Green Valley.

"You really don't need a lot of special ingredients to make your own Hot Oil Hair Pack," Kim told me. "We formulate beautiful mixtures here, but at home it's fine to use just two oils in combination, or only one. Jojoba oil is ideal, but you can even use olive oil from the pantry, if there's nothing else."

You may not have a willow tree swayed by desert breezes, but you probably do have a little extra olive oil somewhere in the house. And four hand towels. And a love of luxurious things.

That's all you'll need. This can be an experience just for you, or you can enjoy it with a partner.

HOT OIL HAIR PACK

Step by Step

1. Rinse the hair first, or moisten with a spritz bottle.

2. Massage a tablespoon or two (depending on the length and bulk of the hair) of jojoba oil or olive oil into the hair and scalp for fifteen minutes. If you have it, rub a few drops of peppermint essential oil into the hair before you start the massage.

3. Layer four hot hand towels over the hair, wrapping them around and around one at a time, making sure to enclose every strand.

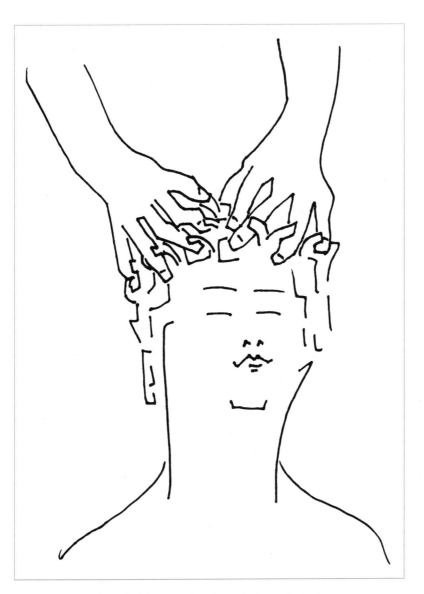

Step 2: Massage the oil gently into the hair.

4. If you're treating yourself, simply recline in a lounge chair or on your bed—with a towel under your headdress, of course. For a partner, spend fifteen minutes massaging the face, neck, arms, hands, and then feet. (See Chapter 8 for the appropriate massage techniques.)

5. Thoroughly rinse the oil mixture out of the hair, using a gentle, natural shampoo and conditioner. You can do this for yourself in the shower, or have your partner lean over the sink. If you're feeling adventurous and have a lounge chair outside, you may try rinsing your partner's hair while they're still lying down. Pour lukewarm water over the scalp from a pitcher, lather with shampoo, then pour more water and condition the hair. The feeling of having your hair washed while lying down is usually the most pleasurable part of going to the stylist. Add it to your repertoire of royal treatments at home!

6. Towel dry. Comb or brush the hair, enjoying its new silkiness and body.

After the Hot Oil Hair Pack, I sat for a few moments in the relaxation area, sipping lime water while awaiting the next appointment. Although my head had been taken care of, my feet were still crying out after the long desert hikes we'd been taking.

A few minutes later I was led to another room, where Marianne greeted me. First, she had me soak my feet in a hot foot bath that had vibrating nubs on the bottom to stimulate the soles. In the meantime my hands were immersed in a mint paraffin bath and then wrapped up in insulated warming gloves. Taking one foot out of the water at a time, she cleaned and trimmed the cuticles, burnished the rough calluses that had been irritated through excess hiking, and filed the nails to smoothness.

Afterward my feet were dipped in the paraffin and wrapped. Marianne then stripped the wax away from my hands and massaged them thoroughly. Ten minutes later she unveiled my feet too and began twenty minutes of reflexology.

Reflexology is a systematic massage of the feet meant to stimulate points corresponding to all the other areas of the body. Marianne was an expert at this, pinpointing certain spots that had been bothering me and explaining how they were related to my liver, lungs, and spine. She applied a cool soothing cream at the end, and when she was finished, my feet were completely pain free and ready for another desert excursion.

MINI-REFLEXOLOGY ROUTINE

The art and science of reflexology has become quite advanced in recent years, and many people practice it with great skill. The following mini-routine is meant solely as a means for you to nurture yourself, not to treat disease. The diagram should not be used as a diagnostic tool. Hundreds of people have learned similar techniques in the spa workshops I teach all across the country; everyone finds it easy to administer and a delight to receive.

In the diagrams on pages 152 and 153, you can see which parts of the feet correspond to which parts of the body. Use this as a basic guide. Apply gentle yet firm pressure, mostly with the pads of your thumbs, feeling for any tight spots or "crystals" (calcified deposits of toxins) and concentrating there.

This mini-routine can be used during the foot treatments described in this chapter.

Step by Step

1. Start at the top, with the toes, giving each one a good squeeze and a gentle pull. Pay extra attention to the big toe, using your thumb to "walk" little lines all over its surface, thereby stimulating the head, neck, face, and brain reflexes.

2. Use your knuckles to press against the pads of the feet between the toes.

3. Squeeze the balls of the feet from above and below at the same time, using your thumb below and your index finger on top of the foot. Place your finger in the groove between the bones that run lengthwise along the foot. This stimulates the chest and lung area.

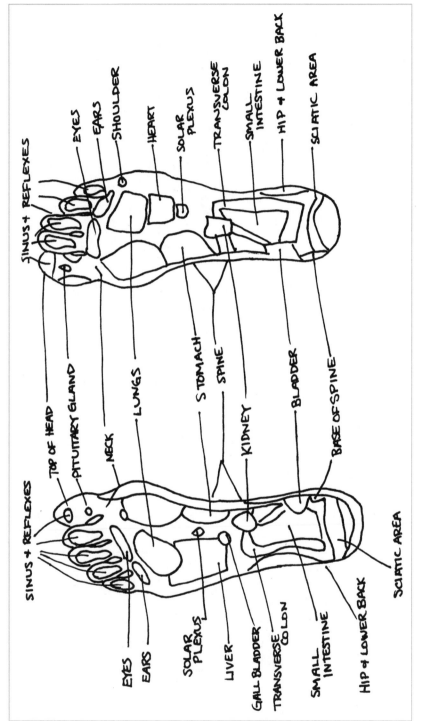

Reflexology Chart: Bottoms of feet

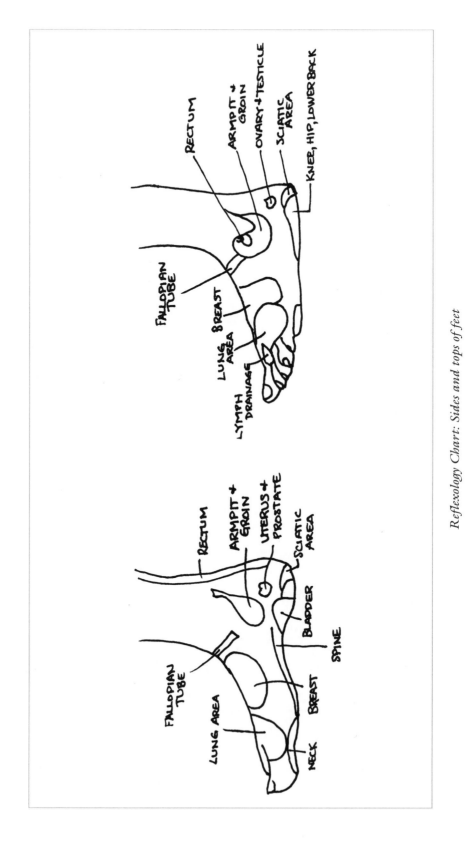

Reflexology Chart: Sides and tops of feet

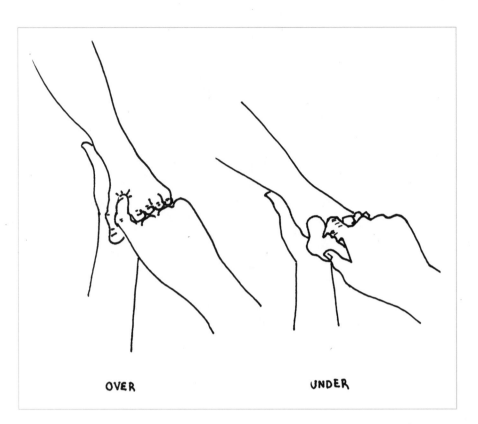

OVER

UNDER

Step 3: Squeeze the balls of the feet from above and below simultaneously.

4. Putting both thumbs on the sole, pointing up toward the toes, "spread" the thumbs apart out toward the edges of the foot while squeezing at the same time.

5. Pinch all over the bottom of the heel, pulling and twisting the taut flesh there firmly, but making sure not to hurt.

6. Inch the tip of your thumb up along the arch of the foot from the heel to the big toe, stimulating the reflex for the spine.

7. Use the tips of your fingers to make little circles all around the inner and outer anklebones.

8. Make circles on the sides of the heels.

9. Squeeze up the back of the Achilles tendon and calf with your cupped palm.

10. Finish with gentle kneading and smoothing-out strokes over the whole foot.

Note: Be careful when performing reflexology on pregnant women because certain points near the ankles are said to stimulate premature labor by affecting the ovaries or uterus. To be safe, avoid the ankles and heels entirely, or choose not to perform reflexology on someone whom you know to be pregnant.

FOOT TREATMENT

You Will Need:

To create your own divine foot treatment, you'll need a place to soak your feet (bathtubs do nicely), nail clippers and files, a cuticle tool, two hot towels, and some skin lotion.

Step by Step

1. Soak your feet in hot water for five minutes, using a foot bath if you have one or simply sitting at the edge of the bathtub. Add some bath salts and a couple of drops of peppermint essential oil for stimulation, if you'd like.

2. While one foot is still soaking, clip and file the nails of the other, cleaning the cuticles too. Repeat for the other foot.

3. Dry the feet off, and wrap each one in a hot towel that has been sprinkled with your favorite essential oil. The hot towels replace the paraffin dip used at Green Valley and many other spas. The deeply penetrating heat of high-quality paraffin is a marvelous tool for any home spa, though, and the price for a foot-sized bath can be reasonable. (See Appendix A.)

The Royal Treatment

4. While the feet are wrapped, take a few minutes to rub some lotion into your hands. Work on your fingernails a little too, applying some polish if it suits your mood.

5. Unwrap one foot at a time, bringing it up to your lap, and spend ten minutes on each, performing the Mini–Reflexology Routine.

6. Finish with a light application of skin lotion to each foot. This is a perfect time to apply toenail polish if you wish.

PARTNER'S FOOT TREATMENT

You'll need the same ingredients as before, with four hot towels this time.

1. One of the most luxurious sensations we can experience is having our feet washed by somebody else. It's an archetypal tradition that stretches back to biblical times. As you begin, place your partner's feet in a hot bath for her, lifting the feet up yourself and gently guiding them into the water. Then, as you wash each foot, take special care and go slowly, swirling a washcloth sensuously around the ankle, between the toes, and over the arch.

2. Lift one foot at a time out of the bath, clipping and filing the nails. Use a cuticle tool if you have one, but it is not absolutely necessary. The important thing is the attention and care you give.

3. Wrap each of your partner's feet in a steaming hot towel as you finish with it.

4. Using skin lotion or massage oil, perform a three-to-five-minute massage on each hand. (See page 90.) Wrap each hand in a hot towel as you finish with it.

5. Unwrapping one foot at a time, perform the ten-minute Mini–Reflexology Routine. You won't need any massage oil

for this step because skin-to-skin friction is appropriate for re-flexology.

6. Unwrap the hands.

7. Finish with a soothing and luxurious application of lotion to the feet.

The Right Books

Richard Hill, spa director at Green Valley, knows the importance of providing the right kind of literature for his guests. For years, he has worked at building the selection of books in the spa's shop. Volume by volume, he has sought out the most inspirational and educational choices, and his work seems to have paid off. There is seldom a time when one of his guests is not perusing the shelves.

"Along with our great food and the treatments, I wanted people to have a resource for spiritual nourishment also," says Richard. "We're taking care of more than just the body here."

True to his word, Richard presented me with a volume during my stay, *A Guide for the Advanced Soul,* and I began reading it immediately. In this way the experience of Green Valley was augmented; the body was worked by hiking, rock climbing, classes, and weight training; we were given the royal treatment from head to toe in the spa services area; *and* the spirit was uplifted through the wisdom contained in the Right Books.

Some other popular titles on the Green Valley shelves include: *The Prophet* by Kahlil Gibran, *A Natural History of Love* and *A Natural History of the Senses* by Diane Ackerman, *The Celestine Prophecy* by James Redfield, the Talmud, the Bible, books about the Dalai Lama and Mahatma Gandhi, *Body Mind* by Ken Dyctwald, all the books by Deepak Chopra, all the books by Carlos Casteneda, *Wherever You Go, There You Are* by Jon Kabat-Zinn, and *A Course in Miracles.*

Your mission: Create your own inspirational library. Reserve a shelf or two someplace in your home *exclusively* for books about health, personal growth, spiritual development, consciousness raising, relationship nurturing, grooming, diet, and physical excellence.

As you wander through bookshops, keep an image of your special library in the back of your mind, and be ready to pick up a book if it strikes you. You'll be amazed at how quickly your collection will grow. Within months you'll have a solid body of reference and wisdom that will refresh you on a daily basis. The words of others reveal their trials and tribulations, their triumphs and recommendations, a treasure of possible paths to follow while you're making your own way toward the challenging goal of optimal health and well-being.

Keep these shelves special. If they're part of an already existing bookshelf, make sure the entire shelf is reserved for your "spa volumes." Or if you have the space, you can build or purchase a couple of shelves specifically for this purpose. Others in your family or perhaps friends who visit will take note. Many may ask to borrow from your collection. All will be inspired by your example. And you'll have your favorite selections right there, easy to find, whenever you want them.

Add Color to Your Days

Color is a focus of attention at the Green Valley Spa. Every day has its own special color scheme. Carole Coombs has worked with an in-depth system of color analysis to create her spa's unique ambience. You too can study books about the intricate effects of color and how different colors reflect the energy centers within our own bodies (called *chakras*).

But as a simple beginning for your own home spa, try working with what you already know. We all realize that different colors affect us differently. Red is for when we're feeling aggressive, bright, outgoing, and passionate. Blue is for the subtler moods of introspection, reflection, and compassion. Green gets us in tune with nature, mellowing us into the world of living things—trees, plants, the sea. Yellow is for simple sunny happiness, orange for a warm inner glow. Using this type of basic color awareness consciously is a big step toward harmonizing yourself with your environment, which is one of the main goals of any spa experience.

COLOR THERAPY

You can create a color theme for your own day in a number of different ways. To begin, in the morning, choose a specific color for that day, and then *go for it* completely by centering the entire theme of that day around the color. You may be surprised by the reactions you get from those around you.

Some things you can do with your chosen color:

- Make a centerpiece for the dining table using plants, flowers, art, glassware, or just pieces of construction paper.
- Squeeze pieces of fruit that match your color into your drinking water.
- Make a bath with your color—for example, sprinkle rose petals in your bath, if the color of the day is pink or rose.
- Buy food that color at the grocery store. Be creative—eggplants for purple, blackberries for black, potatoes for beige!
- In your journal, write down everything you can think of about that color. How does it make you feel? What is your history with it throughout your life?
- Wear something (or everything) that color—a dress, jewelry, a hat.
- Place a colored piece of material (silk works nicely for this purpose) over the lampshades in your room to create the mood of your chosen color.

- Think of a gift you can buy that glows with your chosen color, then give it to someone you love.

For more information:

Amber, Reuben. *Color Therapy.* Santa Fe: Aurora Press, 1983.

Byers, Dwight C. *Better Health with Foot Reflexology.* St. Petersburg, Fla.: Ingham Publishing, 1983.

Ingham, Eunice. *Stories the Feet Can Tell/Have Told Through Reflexology.* St. Petersburg, Fla.: Ingham Publishing, 1984.

"To become delightful, happiness
must be tainted with poison."
—*Georges Bataille*

❧ *Chapter 13* ❧
THE PLEASURE
LIES WITHIN

During my travels over the past year, whenever I met people on planes or on buses or waiting in lines and told them what I was doing, I usually noticed a moist gleam of envy in their eyes. Writing a book about spas? Receiving luxurious treatments at all these wonderful places and writing about them? What could be better? I smiled and politely agreed with them, but inside I knew about the other side of the glamour—the missed flights and nights spent away from my wife and the endless phone calls to public relations people, ironing out details, overnighting press kits, constantly changing plans up to the last minute. Life was not just a bowl of cherry-scented aromatherapy oil.

I reached my apex of frustration when I was trying desperately to get aboard a cruise ship in Alaska to sample their spa and write about it. For several weeks I maintained a constant dialogue with the cruise line's headquarters, but the public relations director was never in a position to give me a firm answer. The night before I had to leave for the cruise, I still did not know for sure if

I was going to be allowed on. In what I thought to be an act of proactive self-assertion, I decided to fly to Alaska anyway and take my chances.

That night I came down with food poisoning. I was very sick. But still determined to pursue my goal, I took the early-morning flight across the country and then the connecting flight up to Juneau. I caught a van to the dock. I spent several hours talking to everyone on the ship who might be able to help me. The public relations director was not in the office that day. Nothing could be done without the public relations director's authorization.

So, my stomach still in knots, my face green, after a miserable transcontinental journey, I walked off the ship with my suitcase in hand. Instead of a five-star luxurious ocean liner, my abode that night was the last available room in Juneau, in an old boarding house, with the sounds of traffic from a local diner wafting up to my window all night long. Around midnight I heard the deep mysterious sound of the cruise ship's horn as it passed out the straits to the sea, leaving me behind.

While my stomach slowly regained its composure, I spent the entire next day on the phone trying to figure out what to do next. Finally I found a seat on a flight back as far as Seattle that night. When I arrived, every hotel I called was already booked. The only vacancy I could find was in a tiny motel a couple miles from the airport, and they only had one room left. The young lady behind the reception desk took one look at me, and an expression of pity filled her large blue eyes. "You look exhausted," she said, "but don't worry. This is our special deluxe suite that you're getting, for the same price as a regular room!"

"What makes it deluxe?" I asked her, unable to keep an edge of sarcasm out of my voice as my eyes glanced over the cheap unadorned lobby.

"It's got a Jacuzzi!" she said.

Sure enough, the room did have a Jacuzzi. Upon first entering the room, I tried for a minute to resist the pull to Conscious Pleasure. I wanted to wallow for a while longer in my state of self-pity and the feeling that I'd been neglected by other people. But when I turned on those jets and poured in some essential oils and lowered myself into the tub in that modest motel near the airport, every last vestige of sickness and frustration left me, and an important lesson finally sank in for me in a very personal way.

The "spa" does not exist out there someplace aboard a fantastic cruise ship navigating the glacial fjords of Alaska. The real spa is inside your heart, in a Jacuzzi overlooking a parking lot in the suburbs of the town you live in or are just visiting. The real spa is inside you.

THE EMERGENCY JACUZZI

Wherever you are, whatever you're doing, the next time you find yourself in a state of stress or self-recrimination, *stop* what you're doing, find the nearest bathtub, fill it with hot-as-you-can-stand-it water, and plunge in. If the tub has Jacuzzi jets attached to it, so much the better, but this is by no means a necessity.

The important thing is for you to transform whatever negative emotions you're experiencing at the moment into something positive that you can use to improve your life and the lives of those you love. The most likely sensation you'll have, if this exercise is handled correctly, is one of gratitude. You'll be so grateful for the things that *are* going right in your life that the few minor inconveniences you're experiencing will pale in comparison. You may also have a sensation of humor—suddenly, as you soak there in your tub, you'll be able to look at yourself with just the slightest wry twist in your grin. What's the big deal anyway? What were you all worked up about?

A quick soak, at the crucial moment, can often save hours or even days of impending negativity from taking place.

As you exit the tub and towel yourself dry, think of the positive steps you can take to improve whatever situation you find yourself in. Then, one step at a time, preferably after you've gotten dressed, head in that direction.

Chapter 14

YOUR NOSE KNOWS— THE JOYS OF AROMATHERAPY

Meadowood Resort and Spa, Napa Valley, Saint Helena, California

Napa Valley's vineyards stretch out far and symmetrical on either side of Highway 29, north of San Francisco. The wineries that dot the roadside are all cool stone and wood, with expensive art in quiet side rooms, statuary on the lawns, and soft-spoken, cultivated people leaning toward each other everywhere you look, discussing the lore of the grape.

On the eastern rim of the valley arcs the Silverado Trail, where tranquil lanes depart the main thoroughfare and disappear up into moss-covered boulders, silent towering redwoods, and magnificent private homes. One of these lanes, marked only by a tiny blue sign, leads to the Meadowood resort, a sanctuary tucked away from the bustle of weekend visitors, with a private golf course, a croquet lawn, a gourmet restaurant, and of course a first-class spa.

I traveled there in late autumn, when the vines had all turned russet and amber, like the foliage of New England. What lured me, besides the beauty and exclusiveness of the resort (and admittedly, a love for the fine wines found so abundantly in the valley), was word of a legendary aromatherapy treatment given by the staff, a treatment unheard of at other properties. The Chardonnay Massage promised to be an experience unlike that found anywhere else, and I was eager to learn more about it.

The spa building itself is nestled snugly amid boulders and pines, a clean wooden structure painted white and gray. The day I arrived was crystal clear, and the building glowed in its socket of the forest. Steam rose from the warmed waters of the hot tubs and pools outside.

Inside, near the reception desk, several shelves were stacked high with bottles of the spa's signature Chardonnay Massage cream. I was immediately drawn to them to learn what was in store for me in one of the treatment rooms hidden down the hallway.

Grapes of all kinds pull at people in the valley, as if they were exuding a gravitational field all their own. Millions of people have taken the drive up Highway 29, magnetized by the irresistible attraction of the tiny round fruits. How, I wondered, would it be possible to incorporate their magic into a spa treatment?

After a leisurely sauna and shower, I headed to treatment room number 3 to find out. I was greeted by Jeanie, a massage therapist on staff, who produced a bottle of the Chardonnay lotion and explained to me finally what the mystique was all about.

"The grapes used to make Chardonnay wine are known for their moisturizing and nutritive qualities," said Jeanie. "In fact, this has been known for a long time. Aristocrats in the French monarchy used to take advantage of their privileged positions, and the ladies of the court often bathed in vats of crushed Chardonnay grapes. What we've tried to do here at the spa is re-create that experience, but just make it a little less messy!"

Jeanie left the room for a moment while I slipped out of my robe and lay down upon the massage table. The first sensation I felt was warmth. A special full-length heating pad was tucked beneath the sheets. When Jeanie came back into the room, she warmed some of the lotion between her palms and began a thorough massage. But first she started me out with a whiff of the rich emollient lotion. It had been imbued with the essence of Chardonnay grapes.

"Do you like it?" she asked. "It took a long time for our supplier to get those grapes into the lotion, but he finally got it right, I think."

"I think you're right," I told her. Smelling the lotion was like catching a subtle trace of a great vintage. It reminded me of experiences I'd had in the region's tasting rooms, where the rich complex bouquet of each bottle floats up to your nose with an ancient pleasing familiarity. Those French aristocrats knew what they were doing. For the next hour the sole purpose of my existence was to be an effective sponge and soak up the healing, moisturizing essence of the grapes while Jeanie kneaded and plied my skin, working the lotion in.

During my stay at Meadowood, I received yet another treatment based on the principles of aromatherapy, which is the therapeutic use of essential oils distilled from the leaves, roots, flowers, bark, nuts, and fruits of plants from all around the world.

This second treatment was an aromatherapy massage using a specially prepared combination of oils called the Balancing Blend because it was intended to balance my body and mind. It worked. After being balanced with the special blend and moisturized with the Chardonnay, I walked out of the spa feeling uplifted and renewed.

Aromatherapy treatments at spas have a tendency to do that to a person, and that is why they are becoming more and more popular today. Treatments based on aromatherapy principles were started long before the French monarchs used vats of crushed grapes. For centuries aromatherapy has been a traditional part of the healing arts. Many ancient cultures, such as the Egyptian, Chinese, Greek, and Indian, developed extensive healing systems based on herbs and essential oil extracts.

During the time of the plague in Europe, those people who worked most closely with essential oils, such as priests and pharmacists, seemed to be spared from contracting the pestilence. Right up until the last century doctors knew and utilized the power of plants extensively. In this century it was the French who made this power a household name. The French, in fact, coined the word *aromatherapy* in the 1930s, and in modern France today doctors often prescribe aromatherapy treatments for their patients. An extensive network of natural pharmacies throughout the country has the oils available for purchase.

When teaching spa therapy workshops, I include a half-hour presentation of some of the best and most useful aromatherapy oils used in spas today. I pass sixteen tiny blue bottles around the room. (Clear bottles are avoided because they allow too much light to enter, which spoils some of the more sensitive oils.) As I describe the attributes of each oil, participants sniff to their heart's content, and by the end of the presentation, many of them experience sensations of giddiness, overwhelmed by the power of the aromas.

Aromatherapy oils and treatments should not be taken lightly. They have the power to heal—and to upset the body's balance if they are not used wisely. One associate of mine added some peppermint oil to the bath of her young son when he came down with the flu. An aromatherapist had recommended just a few drops in the water in order to stimulate circulation and help the boy purge his system. His mother did not know that pouring in half a bottle would be too much of a good thing, and she ended up having to snatch the boy from the water and rub him vigorously with a towel for twenty minutes to warm him up again. Even in the warm bath, the oil's cooling effects caused him to feel cold.

Peppermint is one of the oils included in the spa workshop. When it is passed around, I instruct students to place just the faintest dab on each temple. This has the immediate effect of creating alertness and opening the eyes wider, excellent for people on a long-haul drive or studying late into the night. Each oil has its

Chart of Essential Oils

Oil	Properties
Cedar	Reduces fluids in body tissues, diuretic. Warming in baths.
Clary sage	Balances female hormones. Good for scalp problems.
Eucalyptus radiata	Excellent for lungs, respiratory system. Muscle tonic.
Geranium rose	Balances the skin by effecting sebum. Balances emotions too.
Juniper	Calming and purifying.
Lavender	Antibacterial (first-aid kit in a bottle). Calming. Good for skin.
Lemongrass	Stimulates digestion. Antiseptic, detoxifies lymph. Uplifting.
Orange	Mood elevator.
Peppermint	Stimulates alertness. Good for headaches, colds.
Pine	Painkiller. Natural deodorant.
Rose	Excellent for the skin.
Rosemary	Hair tonic. Astringent. Good for oily skin.
Sandalwood	Grounding and relaxing. Spiritually uplifting. Aids aging skin.
Tea tree	Antiseptic, antifungal, antibacterial. Good for the skin.
Vetiver	Grounding and calming.
Ylang ylang	Aphrodisiac. Relieves tension/stress. Balances dry skin.

own particular use. For your information, I've included the list of oils from the spa workshop here. It covers only a fraction of available essential oils, but they are the most widely used. For information about dozens of other oils, refer to the books listed at the end of the chapter.

When purchasing aromatherapy oils, make sure that they are either organically grown or "wildcrafted," which means that they are picked where they grow naturally in the wild all over the world. Remember not to buy oils in clear bottles. Usually you get what you pay for with aromatherapy, and the less expensive brands tend to be synthetically produced. It's better to buy one or two high-quality bottles than an entire set of drugstore-brand oils. (For a good source of the best oils, see Appendix A.)

Aromatherapy oils are the distilled essence of life itself. The plants that the oils come from are among the most basic forms of life on the planet, receiving energy directly from the sun and distributing it up through the food chain. The precious liquid found in each bottle is so concentrated that it should rarely be used more than a few drops at a time, and few oils should be applied directly to the skin. Instead, you should dilute them in what are called "carrier oils," which can then be used for massage and other therapeutic purposes.

Carrier Oils

- Jojoba oil: Actually a liquid wax, jojoba oil is highly emollient. It contains nutrients that feed the skin and regulate its functions, and it is easily absorbed. Ideal for all skin types, it also conditions and restores health to hair.

- Apricot kernel oil: Light but not thin, apricot kernel oil is very conditioning to the skin. It is a popular ingredient in natural skin care.

- Sweet almond oil: Ideal to use as a base massage oil because it is light and easily absorbed. It is one of the oldest of all oils used for cosmetic purposes.

- Grapeseed oil: Light, exceptionally fine, quickly penetrating, and odorless, this oil is recommended as a facial oil to cleanse and tone oily skin.

- Avocado oil: High in vitamin content, nourishing to the skin.

- Sesame oil: Helps to filter the ultraviolet rays when exposed to the sun. Its small molecular structure allows easy absorption. Favored by Ayurvedic practitioners for its healing properties, it is also considered to be an antiseptic.

- Wheat-germ oil: Rich in vitamins A, B, C, and E (antioxidants). It is nourishing, helps reinforce and strengthen capillaries and regenerate tissue to promote firmness and elasticity in the skin. For these reasons it is highly recommended for use on stretch marks, partly healed scars and lines around the eyes, and as a facial oil for extremely dry skin.

AROMATHERAPY MASSAGE

It is quite simple to create your own Aromatherapy Massage at home. The most important ingredient is, of course, the oil. My suggestion to you is to go out to your nearest supplier and test the aromas of at least a dozen oils. Mark down which ones seem most pleasant or most powerful. Usually our bodies can tell us what we need. Choose two or three oils, and take them home. Then, when you prepare for your Aromatherapy Massage, use the oil that suits your mood in the moment. Do you want some quiet time with lavender or rose? Or are you and your mate in the mood for the stimulating effects of some ylang ylang? You can add drops of pure essentials into a carrier oil according to the recipe below, or you can purchase a ready-to-use blend. Either way, you will encounter the elemental power of the essential oils as they penetrate your pores and affect you on the deepest levels.

You Will Need:

Approximately twenty-five drops of essential oil

2 ounces of carrier oil

Massage sheets and towels

Blend the essential oil into the carrier oil.

Step by Step

1. First, have your partner inhale a particular oil or blend and see if it is appropriate for the massage this day. Moods change on an hourly basis, and with them the craving for certain scents.

2. Your partner lies face-up first, and the massage routine from Chapter 8 is performed in reverse, starting with the last section and moving backward to the first section. In this way your partner will be able to inhale the aromas better at the beginning of the massage.

3. Pour a teaspoon of the chosen oil into your hand and rub your palms together until the oil is warmed. Then make a tent out of your cupped palms and hold them lightly over your partner's nose, an inch or two away. Instruct him to breathe in deeply of the healing scent and engage in Conscious Pleasure Principle Number 4—Letting Go. The oils will help him eliminate negative thoughts, worries, and stress.

4. Proceed with the head, neck, and face massage, then move down to the shoulders, arms, torso, and so on.

5. When you've finished the hour-long massage, tell your partner to leave the oils on his skin to absorb for at least another hour. This is a great time to sit in a sauna for ten or fifteen minutes, if one is available.

AROMATHERAPY APPLICATIONS

Several simple aromatherapy applications can be used at home. After you've chosen a few favorite essential oils, keep them handy, and you'll be able to cook up a quick mini-treatment on a moment's notice whenever you like.

Aromatherapy Bath

One popular technique used at spas is the Aromatherapy Bath, which is very easy. Simply draw the bath, then add ten drops of essential oils after the tub is full. Agitate the water to disperse the oils. Soak for fifteen minutes.

Compress

Four drops of essential oil are added to half a pint of water in a bowl. For a cold compress, use icy water. For a hot compress, use water as hot as you can stand to touch. Place strips of toweling or linen in the water. Wring out, and place them over the area to be treated.

Shower

Rub your body with the appropriate mixture of essential oils in a carrier base and then shower.

Inhalation

In a bowl of almost boiling water, place six to eight drops of essential oil or a blend. Place a towel over your head, and inhale for five minutes. This can also be done over a sink of steaming water, as in the Herbal Inhalation on page 56.

Vaporization

Place two or three drops of essential oil on a light bulb, to fill a small room with essence.

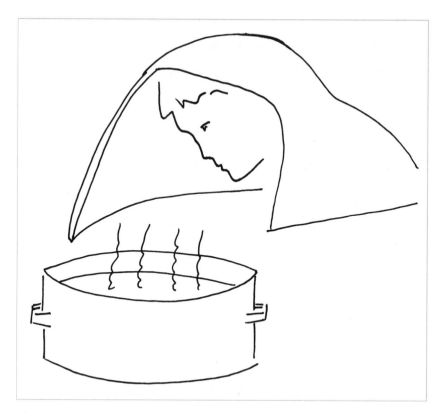

Aromatherapy inhalation

Gargles and Mouthwashes

Add three drops of essential oils to a cup of water and then gargle. Try not to swallow any of the essential oils because they have more powerful reactions internally.

The spa directors who manage the aromatherapy and massage program at Meadowood are Eric and Cathy Chesky, an outdoorsy young couple with healthy complexions and a hands-on attitude. I met up with them when I was leaving the resort after my treatments.

"We strive for a balanced approach to health and wellness," Eric told me. "The therapists here are rewarded for peak performance, and guest satisfaction runs high. We believe that every spa service should be the best we can make it, and we're going to be expanding our services soon because there is such a demand. When you think about it, we have the best ingredients for a great spa experience right here in our backyard: beautiful scenery, high-quality treatments, hiking trails, bicycling, tennis, fitness classes, golf, great food, and of course those Chardonnay grapes!"

This is aromatherapy with a California twist.

For more information about aromatherapy:

Davis, Patricia. *Aromatherapy: An A to Z.* Saffron Walden, Essex, Great Britain: C.W. Daniel Co., 1988.

Lavabre, Marcel. *Aromatherapy Workbook.* Rochester, Vt.: Healing Arts Press, 1990.

Rose, Jeanne. *The Aromatherapy Book.* Berkeley, Calif.: North Atlantic Books, 1992.

Tisserand, Robert B. *The Art of Aromatherapy.* Rochester, Vt.: Healing Arts Press, 1977.

Worwood, Valerie Ann. *The Complete Book of Essential Oils and Aromatherapy.* San Raphael, Calif.: New World Library, 1991.

"Clays, muds, and sand are live mediums
which help generate and maintain life."
—Michel Abehsera
The Healing Clay

❧ *Chapter 15* ❧
FANGO FANDANGO
Camelback Inn, Phoenix, Arizona

A *t some of the most exclusive spas* in the world, people pay premium prices to lie indoors and have mud applied to their bodies, while tennis and golf and the pool are beckoning right outside the door. Why do they do it? Why would anyone voluntarily immerse their body in a tub of thick dark mud? You may have seen pictures of these people dripping in goo or sunk into pits of organic earth. They're usually smiling. Perhaps you thought they know something that you don't. Or, conversely, that you're much smarter than they are. After all, you wouldn't spend good money to get dirty. Right?

The captions below the pictures of people in mud say this is the latest in beauty and indulgence. But why? What's happening for them that couldn't happen for you if you were to simply walk into your backyard with a shovel, spray some water on the ground, and start digging?

The answer is—plenty. Unless you happen to live on a volcanic mountain or on the edge of a spa lake, that is.

Mud is mud is mud, until you start talking about those special muds called fangos and therapeutic clays. The reason that fancy people have slathered themselves with the stuff for hundreds of years is that it actually *does* something for them.

I received my mud initiation at the Doral Spa, while I was a therapist there. Our specialty was coating clients with ash-colored fango mud from the slopes of a volcano in Italy. Mud has a long and illustrious history in Italy, dating back to the first century A.D., when Pliny recorded the use of fango mud packs from the thermal ponds of Battaglia, in northern Italy, to treat arthritis and rheumatism. In recent years other types of muds have become popular in spas as well. Muds in general are called *peloids,* and using them therapeutically is called *peliotherapy.* They fall into the following three categories:

Fango	Volcanic muds
Moor	Muds from inland spa lakes
Clay	From mineral-rich areas, usually high in bentonite

Muds work in two different ways. First, if they are applied warm or used in a bath, they are great heat conductors, and the minerals within them are transmitted directly into the body through the skin. Second, as they dry, they have powerful drawing properties, pulling impurities from the system. The bentonite in some clays is an especially powerful drawing agent.

In search of a world-class peliotherapy of my own, I traveled to the Camelback Inn in Scottsdale, Arizona. There, in a warmed inner room, I reclined upon a specially built table beneath three glowing infrared lights as my body was prepared for a Southwest Adobe Clay treatment.

"This will help get those pores open so the clay can do its work," said Larry, the seasoned spa technician performing the treatment. He was in his seventies, and he worked hard, scrubbing my dead skin cells away with a loofah cloth. Larry is part of a large group of older technicians who choose to work in spas because of the healthful and low-stress environments found there. His clear blue eyes, ruddy skin, and steady hands bespoke a lifestyle that many of the guests he treated would do well to imitate. "This spa job is something I do incognito," he told me with a wink. "My real passion is golf."

After he had prepared my skin, Larry applied some watered-down clay to my back and legs in a thin mask and let the lights begin to dry it. He repeated the procedure on the front of my body, strong fingers dipping into the grainy clay paste and swirling it over my skin. Then he placed a thin gauzy sheet over me.

"That'll keep you warm enough, but let the clay dry at the same time," said Larry. "It'll draw out those impurities. The clay comes from the southwestern deserts out here, so it's like you're getting purged by Mother Nature herself. Folks really like this treatment, once they take the time to slow down and enjoy it."

Slowing down to enjoy it—that was the secret. I closed my eyes, sinking into the sensations of warmth and the tingling tautness of the clay on my skin as it began to dry. This was a time for Conscious Pleasure Principle Number 5—Immersion. Taking a few deep breaths, I let go of the rest of the world, savoring the little healthy piece of it I was experiencing at the moment.

After the clay had dried for twenty minutes, Larry helped me up and led me to a Swiss shower, which is a stall with high-powered shower heads aimed at you from all directions. The forceful stream jetted away the clay mask. After I had toweled off, Larry applied a liberal amount of juniper/sage massage oil and suggested I sit in the sauna for a few minutes to let the effects melt their way into my body. I followed his recommendation.

Judy Snow, assistant spa director at Camelback, believes in the healing power of the treatments given there. "We always tell people to take it easy after their appointments and allow time for the effects to settle in," she told me. Judging by the number of people lounging poolside in spa robes, her advice seems to be heeded. I joined the other guests in the shade near the water, pondering the presence of mud in my life.

In my bathroom for many years now a picture has hung showing me and some friends covered from head to foot in mud. It was taken while I was teaching mud therapy to my class at a massage school in Miami. Everyone remembers that day as the best time we had all semester. The truth is that mud is fun. There's even a spa known as Club Mud in southern California, where people go to wallow in a natural mud pit on the property and bake afterward in the sun. It's called Glenn Ivy, and it's a great place to go with friends or family. And the mountain town of Calistoga, in northern California, is pocketed with more than a dozen spas specializing in mud therapy. Also, most of the mini-spas you'll find in cities and towns all across the country have a moor mud facial or body treatment to offer.

Mud is out there waiting for you. If you never have the chance to visit a spa to have professionals apply mud to your body, you can experiment at home. It might be a little messy, but that's where your spa towels come in handy. The following seven treatments are easy to do, very good for you, and you may just end up having some fun along the way. Create your own Club Mud!

MUD OR CLAY WRAP

In my spa workshops I usually limit the coverage of mud to just the back. Without a wet room, this treatment can get messy. But if you are close enough to your shower at home, there is no reason you can't perform a full-body Mud Wrap. Just make sure to glance at yourself in the mirror before rinsing off; the laugh that you'll have is as therapeutic as any minerals in the mud itself.

Preparation

Of course, you're going to need a little mud to do any of the mud treatments. It's easier to find than you might think. In Appendix A you'll find sources for ordering mud, or you can purchase it from most beauty supply stores, as well as many salons and department stores.

Use dark-colored towels while doing these treatments. Some muds can stain lighter-colored fabrics. There's no need to be concerned with your plumbing, though, because all of these products drain easily, without clogging, and they're completely biodegradable.

Most spa products feel better if they are applied warm. This is doubly true for muds and clays. If they are not warmed sufficiently before the treatment, quite likely the only response you'll get from your partner is one of unpleasant surprise. To heat mud, a double-boiler setup is ideal, allowing steam to surround the receptacle containing the product. If you aren't set up for that, add a couple of tablespoons of extra water to the bottom of a pan before placing the mud inside, and then heat it on low for fifteen minutes. In general, you can make the consistency a little more watery than you'd think: the mud heats faster that way, and it ends up spreading on the skin much more easily.

Lay a wool blanket out on the floor or massage table. On top of the blanket place a sheet of plastic. This is going to be discarded after the wrap, so don't go to any expense over it. A large plastic garbage bag cut in half with scissors does nicely for this purpose. As an alternative, you can use an old sheet. You'll have to launder it separately after the treatment, and it may not be very presentable afterward, but some people prefer to avoid the feeling of plastic on their skin.

Step by Step

1. Make sure the room you're in is warm. Have your partner lie face-up on the plastic wrap or sheet. Lightly exfoliate her skin with a loofah or dry skin brush. Have her turn facedown and repeat the procedure.

2. Apply warmed mud to her back, either with your fingers or with a natural-bristle paintbrush, not slapping the mud on

thick but rather just barely covering the chosen area with a thin layer of color. Ask her to turn over, and repeat the application on the front.

3. For a remineralizing treatment, spritz or sprinkle purified water on all areas covered with mud. In this manner the mud will stay moist, and your partner will continue to absorb minerals and nutrients from it. Wrap your partner cocoon fashion with the plastic sheet first and then the blanket. Make sure she's comfortable. She can remain wrapped for twenty to twenty-five minutes.

4. As an alternative, if you desire a detoxifying treatment, leave your partner unwrapped. Make sure she stays warm enough, and check every few minutes to see how the mud is drying on the skin. Ten to fifteen minutes after she feels a sensation of "tautness," send her to the shower.

5. Shower the mud off. You'll have to give your partner a loofah scrub or brush in order to get all the clingy mud particles to come away. While she showers off, clean up the sheet and blanket.

6. Pat the skin with a towel, but there's no need to dry completely. Now is the time to lock in the minerals and moisture by applying moisturizing lotion or even (if your partner is lucky) by massaging in a high-quality oil, using the Spa Massage techniques from Chapter 8.

MUD FACE PACK

Moor mud is especially good for this treatment. One and a half ounces will be sufficient, diluted with a tablespoon of water to make application easier. Moor mud comes from the nutrient-rich bottom of thermal spring-fed lakes and is therefore filled with bio-dynamic life-giving substances. Several brands are readily available at cosmetic counters and in beauty supply stores. Your face will drink it in.

Step by Step

1. Remove any makeup, then cleanse the face with a toner.

2. Apply a mask in a thin layer, spreading the warmed mud with your fingers or a small cosmetic brush.

3. Keep the mask moist by spritzing or sprinkling with water.

4. For fifteen minutes, see if you can concentrate on Conscious Pleasure Principle Number 4—Letting Go. Ideally, sit quietly by yourself for this quarter hour, knowing that you are the most important person in your life for these moments, nobody else.

5. Wash off with water over the sink. If you're giving this treatment to a partner, you can use two or three hot towels to remove the mask while she is lying down.

6. Apply a final hot towel to the face, and press firmly for thirty seconds. As you lift it away, make sure to wipe up any last remnants of mud.

7. Gently massage the face for a few minutes with an emollient lotion. (See page 92 for face massage techniques.)

MUD OR CLAY BATH

This is a great way to soak minerals directly into the skin. Heat from the bath water makes pores more open for absorption. Place half a cup of powdered clay in a hot bath (95 to 100 degrees). Stir it in thoroughly. When you submerge, try to visualize nutrients coming straight from the Earth into your body, replenishing you. A few moments of meditation are definitely in order for this "Earthy" treatment. Be careful not to stay too long, because after more than twenty or thirty minutes, the effect of hot water and clay together can end up drying your skin.

SPORT FANGO

One of the best things you can do for yourself, if you've had muscle strain caused by a minor sports injury or are suffering from repetitive stress syndrome, is to pack the affected area with warmed mud. Try including a few drops of essential oil in the mixture too. Peppermint is ideal for this purpose. We used to do this at the Doral Spa for active people coming off the golf course or tennis court. Be careful to warm the mud on low heat, and test it on a finger before applying. Spread the mud thickly (thicker than for the body wrap) on the injured area, and then cover it with a piece of plastic or a moist towel. Wipe off after twenty minutes. If you can get somebody to administer a little Spa Massage directly after the mud application, you'll most likely feel much better the next day.

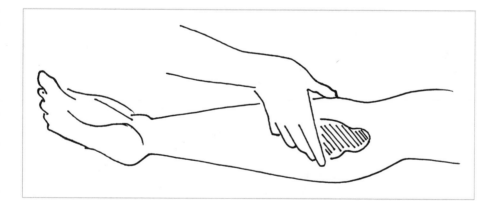

Peppermint oil and warm mud soothe sore muscles.

MUD HAND PACK

When I was managing a team of thirty-five massage therapists at one large spa, we worked eight-hour days doing difficult massage techniques, and we often felt pain in our wrists and fingers. At the end of those long days, we'd gather in the mud preparation room and take turns brushing a thin layer of heated fango onto our aching joints. Then we'd wrap our hands in plastic, keeping them warm for five to ten minutes before washing our fingers off and enjoying the immediate sensations of relief. You can benefit from this too, even if you're not a spa therapist. Those people especially receptive to the pleasures of this simple treatment include secretaries and other professionals who spend a lot of time at the keyboard. Also mechanics, surgeons, seamstresses, and everyone else who depends on their hands at work will find it a godsend. Give it a try.

MUD OR CLAY FOOT SOAK

If you're looking for the quickest way to soak up the benefits of a Mud or Clay Bath but don't want to dirty the tub or towels, try starting with your feet. In a foot bath or bucket, pour two gallons of hot water (100 degrees). Add a quarter cup of powdered clay or moor mud, and stir. Simply dip your feet in for fifteen or twenty minutes. Sit back and relax.

MUD FIRST AID

Besides being a key ingredient in many royal treatment programs, muds and clays have had a long history of use in therapeutic applications as well. Indigenous peoples have known for centuries that the drawing power of muds and clays is perfect for minor insect stings. Have a store of powdered clay handy, and the next time a bee or other pest zaps you or one of the kids, quickly mix up a paste and apply a smidgen directly over the sting. Let it dry in place for half an hour, and then gently wash it away.

For more information about therapeutic muds and clays:

Abehsera, Michel. *The Healing Clay.* New York: Citadel Press, 1994.

Dextreit, Raymond. *Our Earth, Our Cure.* New York: Citadel Press, 1993.

*"The trick with spa food is to take out the fat
but not the flavor, not the enjoyment."*
—Chris Wingate
Executive spa chef

❦ *Chapter 16* ❦

THE TASTE OF HEALTH

PGA Resort and Spa,
West Palm Beach, Florida

W**ith three gourmet restaurants** and their attendant chefs
under her nutritional tutelage, plus a full schedule of national
and international speaking engagements at which she enlightens
the world about healthy eating habits, Cheryl Hartsough, registered dietitian, has become a leading authority on spa foods and spa
dining.

Cheryl is the lead nutritionist at the PGA Resort and Spa in
West Palm Beach, Florida. Thousands of hungry golfers, spa goers,
and vacationers pass into the sphere of her dietary influence each
year, all of whom want to enjoy themselves but at the same time
not feel guilty about it.

At the International Spa and Fitness Association's annual conference, Cheryl has created spa food banquets for more than eight
hundred of the most discriminating palates, and yet she takes time
to counsel guests at the spa one-on-one as well. When those seeking nutritional guidance visit her office at the resort property, they

receive an immediate reminder of what it is they've come to avoid. A large sickly-yellow slab of plasticized lard sits on her desk, for those who would too easily forget who the enemy is.

"This is what five pounds of fat looks like inside your body," Cheryl says, hefting the bulky blob and smiling. "Kind of makes you want to move into a spa for good, doesn't it?" She has red hair, freckles, and a figure that makes guests want to do whatever it is she does to stay in shape. They listen to her straightforward talk about proper diet, and they take the news home with them.

"Spas will always stay low fat, but they don't have to teach deprivation," counsels Cheryl. "Instead, they can teach you how to love and enjoy wholesome food. Many spas are getting away from weight loss, and the spa experience is becoming more about feeling healthy, energized, and nourished rather than losing a few pounds that may come back again later anyway."

I visited Cheryl at the PGA Spa to learn the latest information about spa cuisine. On the way to the dining room we passed through the "waters of the world" spa area, with its hydrotherapy pools and treatment rooms. Although an atmosphere of calm prevailed, the resort was bustling. Hundreds of meals are served in the three restaurants there every day, one of which was voted among the top ten in Palm Beach County. The downstairs dining room is dedicated predominantly to spa cuisine, which means that the items on the menu are prepared with health uppermost in mind. The Italian restaurant and the seafood restaurant serve a regular menu, but several items are highlighted as spa cuisine, and every day the chefs prepare a few spa specialties. They usually sell fast.

"The trick with spa food is to take out the fat but not the flavor, not the enjoyment," says Chris Wingate, the top chef at the seafood restaurant. "You have to fool the mouth. What the taste buds are looking for are the texture and weight of food, along with the taste. So if you can keep the taste consistent, and then provide the texture with a few tricks, your mouth thinks it's eating high-calorie, high-fat food when really it's not."

Chris accomplishes this feat with some amazingly simple techniques. For example, on the night I dined in his restaurant, one spa item offered was sesame-encrusted scallops. Sesame seeds are quite high in fat, and to get around that fact without sacrificing the "feel" of the food, Chris toasted some rice, ground it in a food processor, and mixed it at a ratio of four parts ground rice to one part sesame seeds. The result was a crunchy, satisfying, sesame-tasting dish. I couldn't tell the difference.

"For guests staying at a spa, meals are the highlight of their day," says Cheryl. "Food is like a reward after long hours of aerobics classes, weight lifting, swimming, and sports. People say, 'I've earned this.' And they don't want birdseed. They want something that will nourish tired muscles and refuel their brains."

The secret? According to Cheryl, it's a matter of getting back to nature. "We have our own herb garden here and access to an organic farm nearby. So the food we serve is fresh, with minimal processing. It's important to eat local foods, to make the most of what you have in your area. You won't see any apples on our menu here in Florida, but plenty of citrus. Food that's eaten as close to its origin as possible is the key."

Your Own Spa Menu

The following meals are designed to be used during the three Spa Days described in the next chapter. Cheryl has selected them from the PGA Spa's collected recipes and tailored them to fit with each particular Spa Day. Of course, if you'd prefer, any of the dishes can be prepared and eaten on their own too. You needn't wait until your first full Spa Day to try them out!

Assisting Cheryl in her development of menus is Anne Bramham, a spa treatment expert who specializes in whole-body wellness. She has her own spa training center, called the Bramham Institute, at PGA. I consulted with her about the exact effects of some of the ingredients in these recipes and how they will most benefit you during your home spa program.

When you begin preparing any of these spa dishes, keep these key points in mind:

1. Use foods close to where they were grown whenever possible.
2. "Fool" the mouth with the textures and weights of food.
3. Eat fresh, unprocessed foods whenever you can.

Day One: The Beauty/Pampering Day *(see page 210 for more details)*

Menu items today are chosen to nourish the skin. You will be taking in extra vitamins A (beta carotene) and C, plus silica, which can be found in the skins of fruit. The avocado salsa is rich in essential fatty acids, another skin nourisher. The celery in the apple-pear salad has high natural sodium, which is a "youthing" element for keeping skin hydrated.

Breakfast
2 Banana Bran Muffins
1 fresh whole orange

Lunch
Butternut Squash Soup
Grilled Chicken Caesar Salad

Dinner
Smoked Turkey Quesadilla, with Black Bean Relish
Spa Avocado Salsa

Spa snacks
cantaloupe
Apple-Pear Salad

Banana Bran Muffins

vegetable cooking spray
$^3/_4$ cup boiling skim milk
$^1/_2$ cup unprocessed bran
$^1/_2$ cup regular or quick rolled oats (not instant)
2 cups mashed ripe bananas
2 egg whites
1 cup all-purpose flour
$^1/_4$ cup firmly packed brown sugar
2 tbsp. vegetable oil
2 tsp. baking power
$1^1/_2$ tsp. ground cinnamon
$1^1/_4$ tsp. baking soda
1 tsp. vanilla extract
$^1/_4$ tsp. salt

Preheat oven to 375 degrees F. Spray 12 muffin cups ($2^1/_2''$) with cooking spray or line with paper liners; set aside. In a large bowl stir the milk, bran, and oats; let stand 5 minutes. Add the remaining ingredients; stir just until blended. Spoon into prepared muffin cups, filling $^2/_3$ full. Bake for 25 minutes until toothpick inserted comes out clean.

Makes 12 muffins. Per muffin: calories 137; fat 2.9 g; cholesterol 0 mg; carbohydrate 25 g; protein 3 g.

Butternut Squash Soup

4 cups low-sodium chicken stock, skimmed
$1^1/_2$ lb. fresh butternut squash, peeled, seeded, and cut into chunks
1 lb. green apples, cored and chopped
$^1/_2$ lb. yellow onion (about 2 medium), peeled and chopped
1 tsp. lemon juice
2 sprigs fresh or 1 tbsp. dried rosemary

2 sprigs fresh or 1 tbsp. dried marjoram
$^1/_4$ tsp. salt
$^1/_4$ tsp. black pepper

In a large saucepot or Dutch oven over medium heat, bring all ingredients to a boil. Reduce heat; cover and simmer 30 minutes until squash is tender. In a blender at high speed, puree the mixture in several batches until smooth.

Makes 12 $^3/_4$-cup servings. Per serving: calories 68; fat 0.6 g; cholesterol 0 mg; carbohydrate 15 g; protein 1 g.

Grilled Chicken Caesar Salad

8 cups romaine lettuce, coarsely chopped
40 asparagus tips, blanched and cooled
12 cherry tomatoes, cut in half
2 cups whole-wheat pasta (rotini), cooked
1 cup Spa Caesar Dressing (see below)
2 tbsp. grated Parmesan cheese
4 grilled boneless, skinless chicken breasts
   (5 oz. each), cut into julienne strips

In a large bowl combine the romaine, asparagus, tomatoes, and pasta. Add the dressing and cheese; toss to coat well. To serve: On each of 4 dishes place $^1/_4$ of the salad topped with $^1/_4$ of the chicken. Serve immediately.

Makes 4 servings. Per serving: calories 440; fat 10 g; cholesterol 127 mg; carbohydrate 32 g; protein 54.5 g.

Spa Caesar Dressing

1 cup low-sodium chicken stock or broth, skimmed
$^1/_2$ cup raspberry vinegar
2 tbsp. olive oil
1 tbsp. cornstarch
$^1/_2$ tbsp. water
1 tbsp. fresh chopped or $^1/_2$ tsp. dried herbs

$^1/_2$ tbsp. minced garlic

$^1/_4$ tbsp. sugar

$^1/_2$ cup nonfat sour cream

$^1/_2$ tbsp. anchovy fillets, drained

In a food processor or blender, puree all the ingredients until smooth.

Makes 10 $^1/_4$-cup servings. Per serving: calories 45; fat 3.4 g; cholesterol 5 mg; carbohydrate 3 g; protein 0.5 g.

Smoked Turkey Quesadilla

4 whole-wheat-flour tortillas (8″ each)

$^1/_2$ cup shredded part-skim mozzarella cheese

8 oz. skinless, boneless smoked turkey, diced

2 cups shredded greens

1 cup Black Bean Relish (see below)

$^1/_2$ cup Spa Avocado Salsa (see page 194)

$^1/_2$ cup nonfat sour cream

For each quesadilla: In a 9″ skillet over high heat place a tortilla; sprinkle with 2 tbsp. of the cheese and 2 oz. of the turkey. Cook until the cheese melts; fold in half, and remove from pan. To serve: Cut each quesadilla in thirds. On each of 4 plates place $^1/_2$ cup greens topped with cut quesadilla, $^1/_4$ cup relish, 2 tbsp. salsa, and 2 tbsp. sour cream.

Makes 4 servings. Per serving: calories 345; fat 9 g; cholesterol 66 mg; carbohydrate 34 g; protein 31 g.

Black Bean Relish

1 cup cooked or canned black beans, rinsed and drained

$^1/_4$ cup thawed frozen or vacuum-packed canned
    whole-kernel corn

$^1/_4$ cup diced, seeded tomato

2 tbsp. lime juice

2 tbsp. low-sodium chicken stock or broth, skimmed

1 tbsp. chopped fresh cilantro
1 tbsp. minced garlic

In a small bowl stir all the ingredients until well blended.
Cover and refrigerate at least 1 hour to blend flavors.

Spa Avocado Salsa

4 medium tomatoes, diced
1 large avocado, seeded, peeled, and diced
$1/4$ cup diced red onion
2 tbsp. lemon juice
2 tbsp. chopped fresh cilantro
1 tbsp. minced garlic

In a medium bowl gently stir all the ingredients until combined. Refrigerate at least 1 hour to blend flavors.

Apple-Pear Salad

2 Granny Smith apples, cored and sliced
2 medium pears, cored and sliced
$3/4$ cup sliced celery
$1/4$ cup lemon juice
2 tbsp. raspberry vinegar
2 tbsp. chopped parsley
1 tbsp. olive oil
1 tsp. ground black pepper

In a large bowl gently stir all the ingredients until well coated.
Cover and refrigerate 15 minutes to blend flavors.

Makes 10 $1/2$-cup servings. Per serving: calories 52; fat 1.5
g; cholesterol 0 mg; carbohydrate 10 g; protein 0 g.

You'll be needing extra carbohydrates and B vitamins for exercising your muscles today. Remember not to eat right before your treatments or immediately before exercise. And drink plenty of water—at least two quarts throughout the day.

Breakfast
Bran Crepes with Fruited Cottage Cheese Filling

Lunch
Guava Barbecued Shrimp
Wildberry Cheesecake

Dinner
Spa Rolls
Fusilli Marco Polo
skim milk

Spa snacks
kiwi
orange
Energy Bar

Bran Crepes with Fruited Cottage Cheese Filling

Crepes:
vegetable cooking spray
1 cup whole-wheat flour
3 tbsp. unprocessed bran
$1/8$ tsp. salt
pinch ground cinnamon
1 cup skim milk
1 egg

Filling:
1 1/2 cups 1%-fat cottage cheese
1 1/2 cups Pear, Apple, Raisin Compote (see below)
3/4 cup plain low-fat yogurt
6 tbsp. Fruit Puree, made with strawberries (see page 197)
parsley sprigs for garnish

For crepes: Spray a 6″ nonstick skillet or crepe pan with cooking spray; set aside. In a medium bowl combine the flour, bran, salt, and cinnamon; beat in the milk and egg till smooth. Preheat the skillet over medium-high heat. Spoon 2 tbsp. of the batter into the pan; tilt to spread evenly. Cook until the edges begin to dry; turn, and cook 1 minute more. Turn out onto waxed paper. Repeat with the remaining batter.

For filling: In a medium bowl stir cottage cheese and Compote until well combined. To serve: Place about 1/4 cup filling on each crepe; roll up. On each plate place 2 filled crepes; top with 2 tbsp. yogurt, and drizzle with 1 tbsp. Puree. Garnish with parsley.

Makes 6 servings. Per serving: calories 225; fat 2 g; cholesterol 50 mg; carbohydrate 38 g; protein 13.5 g.

Pear, Apple, Raisin Compote

3 pears, cored, peeled, and diced
3 Granny Smith apples, cored, peeled, and diced
1 1/3 cups golden raisins
1 1/2 cups unsweetened apple juice
2 tbsp. lemon juice or juice of one lemon
1/4 cup honey
1 tsp. ground cinnamon
1 tsp. arrowroot

In a large saucepan over medium heat, cook all the ingredients until of desired consistency, stirring occasionally.

Fruit Puree

1 lb. ripe fruit, peeled, pitted, and cut in pieces, if needed
    (raspberries, strawberries, peaches, plums, figs, apricots,
    or cherries)
$^1/_2$ cup water

In a food processor or blender, place the fruit and water.
Puree for a few seconds or at low speed until slightly chunky.
In a small saucepan over medium-low heat, simmer 5 minutes.
Serve warm or cold.

Guava Barbecued Shrimp

1 lb. large shrimp (16-20), peeled and deveined
$^1/_2$ cup Guava Barbecue Sauce (see page 198)
2 cups cooked cellophane noodles
$^1/_2$ cup julienned red bell pepper
$^1/_2$ cup Pineapple Teriyaki Sauce (see page 198)
4 cups torn salad greens
1 cup Banana Salsa (see page 198)

In a medium saucepan stir the shrimp and Barbecue Sauce; let
stand 30 minutes. Preheat grill or broiler. Lightly drain the
shrimp, reserving the extra Barbecue Sauce. Grill or broil the
shrimp until done, turning constantly. Meanwhile in a large
skillet over medium-high heat, stir-fry the cellophane noodles,
pepper, and Pineapple Teriyaki Sauce until the pepper is ten-
der-crisp. Heat reserved Barbecue Sauce to boiling. To serve:
On each of 4 plates place 1 cup salad greens topped with
$^1/_4$ noodle mixture alongside $^1/_4$ cup Banana Salsa topped
with $^1/_4$ of the shrimp. Just before serving, brush the shrimp
with heated Barbecue Sauce.

Makes 4 servings. Per serving: calories 308; fat 2 g; cholesterol 135 mg; carbohydrate 51 g; protein 19 g.

Guava Barbecue Sauce

$1/4$ cup ketchup
1 tbsp. guava puree
1 tbsp. cider vinegar
$1/2$ tbsp. honey
1 tsp. brown sugar
$1/2$ tsp. jerk seasoning
$1/2$ tsp. vegetable oil

In a small bowl whisk all the ingredients until well blended. Store covered in refrigerator up to 4 weeks. Note: Jerk seasoning is available in the spice section of a supermarket or specialty food store. If not available, substitute Worcestershire sauce, allspice, cinnamon, sugar, garlic powder, scallion, ground pepper, and Tabasco to taste.

Pineapple Teriyaki Sauce

vegetable cooking spray
1 clove garlic, minced
$1/2$ cup unsweetened pineapple juice
$1/2$ cup chopped fresh or canned crushed pineapple
$1/4$ cup lite soy sauce
2 tbsp. chopped fresh or 2 tsp. dried basil
$1/2$ tbsp. cornstarch

Spray a medium saucepan with cooking spray. Add the garlic; cook over medium-high heat 1 minute. Add the remaining ingredients; bring to a boil, stirring. Reduce heat to low; simmer 5 minutes, stirring occasionally.

Banana Salsa

$1/3$ cup diced banana
$1/3$ cup diced, seeded tomato
$1/4$ cup diced red onion

2 tbsp. cider vinegar
1 tbsp. brown sugar
1 tsp. chopped cilantro

In a small bowl gently stir all the ingredients until well combined. Cover and refrigerate a least 1 hour to blend flavors.

Wildberry Cheesecake

Crust:
vegetable cooking spray
$1^1/_2$ cups graham-cracker crumbs
$^1/_4$ cup apple juice with vitamin C

Filling:
2 tbsp. unflavored gelatin
$^1/_2$ cup water
2 cups 1%-fat cottage cheese
1 cup nonfat ricotta cheese
1 pkg. (8 oz.) lite cream cheese (Neufchatel)
$^1/_4$ cup sugar
1 tbsp. vanilla extract
$^1/_2$ cup Fruit Puree, made with strawberries (see page 197)

For crust: Preheat oven to 350 degrees F. Spray a 9" springform pan with cooking spray; set aside. In a medium bowl stir the crumbs and apple juice until well combined. With the back of a spoon, press the crumb mixture evenly into the prepared pan. Bake 5 minutes. Cool.

For filling: In a small saucepan sprinkle the gelatin over the water; let stand 5 minutes to soften. Cook over low heat until dissolved, stirring. Set aside. In a food processor or blender, process the gelatin mixture and the next 5 ingredients until smooth. Stir in the fruit puree. Pour into the prepared crust. Refrigerate at least 2 hours or until set.

Makes 10 servings. Per serving: calories 180; fat 2 g; cholesterol 21 mg; carbohydrate 28 g; protein 12 g.

Spa Rolls

These luscious little rolls require very little effort. Freeze some for later use, if they last long enough!

1 large onion, finely chopped
2 sprigs chopped fresh or 2 tsp. dried rosemary
$^1/_2$ cup dry white wine
$1^1/_2$ cups finely ground whole-wheat flour
$1^1/_2$ cups all-purpose or bread flour
1 cup warm water (125–130 degrees F.)
$1^1/_2$ tbsp. instant fast-acting yeast
$^1/_2$ tbsp. honey
1 tsp. salt

In a small saucepan over low heat, simmer the onion, rosemary, and wine, covered, for 20 minutes. Cool to room temperature. In a large mixer or food processor (with the dough blade attached), combine the remaining ingredients. Mix or process 15 minutes. Remove and knead on a lightly floured surface for 5 minutes until smooth and elastic. Place in a greased bowl; cover and let rise in a warm, draft-free place for 1 hour, until double in size. Punch down; cut into 13 equal portions. Shape into round rolls. Place on lightly greased baking sheets. With your thumb press down the center of each roll; fill with $^1/_2$ tsp. onion mixture. Preheat oven to 375 degrees F. Cover the rolls lightly with a clean towel; let them rise again until double in size. Bake 20 minutes until golden brown.

Makes 13 rolls. Per roll: calories 124; fat 0.6 g; cholesterol 0 mg; carbohydrate 20 g; protein 9 g.

Fusilli Marco Polo

$^1/_2$ cup broccoli florets
4 shiitake mushrooms, cut into julienne strips
$^1/_2$ small onion, cut into julienne strips

1 tsp. minced garlic
1 tsp. virgin olive oil
5 large scallops
$^1/_4$ cup low-sodium chicken stock, skimmed
dash sherry
salt and pepper to taste
$1^1/_2$ cups cooked fusilli

In a large skillet over medium-high heat, sauté the broccoli, mushrooms, onion, and garlic in oil for 3 minutes, stirring. Add the scallops and stock. Cook 5–10 minutes more until scallops are done, stirring. Add the sherry with salt and pepper to taste. Serve over fusilli.

Makes 1 serving. Per serving: calories 425; fat 7 g; cholesterol 25 mg; carbohydrate 69 g; protein 27 g.

Energy Bar

vegetable cooking spray
4 oz. dried apricots, finely chopped
3 cups puffed rice cereal
$1^1/_2$ cups regular or quick rolled oats (not instant)
1 cup puffed wheat cereal
$^1/_2$ cup unprocessed bran
$^1/_2$ cup thawed frozen unsweetened apple juice concentrate
$^1/_2$ cup raisins
$^1/_2$ cup honey
3 tbsp. light corn syrup
2 tbsp. molasses
1 tsp. ground cinnamon
2 tbsp. dry sesame seeds

Preheat oven to 275 degrees F. Spray a 11″ × 7″ baking pan with cooking spray; set aside. In a large bowl with a wooden spoon, mix the apricots and next 10 ingredients for 5 minutes, until well combined. Turn into the prepared pan; flatten with spatula, pushing down hard. Sprinkle with sesame seeds; flatten again. Bake 50 minutes (for chewy texture) to 1 hour. Cool on wire rack 10 minutes. With a very sharp knife cut into 15 bars (5 columns by 3 rows). To store: Tightly wrap each bar individually in foil. Store for up to 1 week. Freeze for longer storage.

Makes 15 bars. Per bar: calories 157; fat 1 g; cholesterol 0 mg; carbohydrate 35 g; protein 2.5 g.

Day Three:
The Detox Day *(see page 214 for more details)*

Try to take a multivitamin/mineral supplement and extra calcium during this Spa Day, because you are going to be consuming no animal products or dairy. You'll do this in order to cleanse your system, and therefore it's a good idea to drink some water as soon as you wake up and continue to drink a total of at least eight glasses by the end of the day.

Breakfast
Tropical Smoothie

Lunch
Chilled Fruit Soup
Garden Pocket Melt

Dinner
Vegetable Harvest Soup
Hot Spinach Salad

Spa snacks
carrot sticks
apple slices
rice cakes

Tropical Smoothie

1 ripe medium banana, frozen and cut into pieces
1 chopped papaya
1 chopped mango
8 ice cubes
$^1/_2$ cup unsweetened pineapple juice
$^1/_2$ cup coconut milk

In a blender combine all the ingredients; blend until smooth.

Makes 4 1-cup servings. Per serving: calories 130; fat 4.5 g; cholesterol 0 mg; carbohydrate 12.5 g; protein 1 g.

Chilled Fruit Soup

30 strawberries, divided
$^1/_2$ medium cantaloupe, peeled and cut into pieces
$^1/_2$ pineapple, peeled and cut into pieces
1 banana, peeled and sliced
$^1/_2$ cup orange juice
1 tbsp. honey
$^1/_2$ cup ginger ale
alfalfa sprouts for garnish
3 coconuts, cut in half, optional
6 mint sprigs, for garnish

Cut 6 of the strawberries into quarters and 18 strawberries into fans; set aside. In a blender combine the remaining 6 strawberries and the cantaloupe, pineapple, banana, orange juice, and honey; blend until smooth. Add the ginger ale. To serve: On each of 6 plates place a bed of alfalfa sprouts; top with a coconut half or soup bowl; fill with $^1/_6$ of the fruit soup. Float 4 strawberry quarters in each bowl. Garnish with a sprig of fresh mint.

Makes 6 servings. Per serving: calories 113; fat 0 g; cholesterol 0 mg; carbohydrate 27 g; protein 2 g.

Garden Pocket Melt

$3/4$ cup oriental vegetables (bok choy, snow peas, bean
   sprouts, zucchini, yellow squash, carrots, red pepper),
   cut into bite-size pieces
2 tbsp. Spa Soy Sauce (see below)
1 medium whole-wheat pita, cut in half crosswise
2 heaping tbsp. nondairy soy cheese, grated
$1/2$ cup Black Bean Relish (see page 193)
3 leaves Bibb lettuce, for garnish
1 leaf radicchio, for garnish
$1/4$ cup alfalfa sprouts, for garnish
2 carrot curls, for garnish

Preheat oven to 350 degrees F. In a medium skillet over
medium heat, sauté the vegetables in the Soy Sauce until most
of the liquid has been evaporated. Remove from heat. In each
pita half place half the vegetables topped with half the soy
cheese. Bake until the cheese melts. To serve: Arrange on a
plate with the Relish and the vegetable garnishes.

   Makes 1 serving. Per serving: calories 337; fat 6 g;
cholesterol 16 mg; carbohydrate 53 g; protein 17 g.

Spa Soy Sauce

5 tbsp. low-sodium vegetable broth
5 tbsp. low-sodium soy sauce
5 tbsp. orange juice
1 tbsp. prepared horseradish
1 tbsp. honey

In a covered container or jar shake all the ingredients until
blended. Store in the refrigerator for up to 2 weeks.

   Makes 8 servings. Per serving: calories 19; fat 0 g;
cholesterol 0 mg; carbohydrate 4 g; protein 0.6 g.

Vegetable Harvest Soup

1 carrot, peeled and diced
1 rib celery, diced
$^1/_2$ medium onion, peeled and diced
1 tbsp. minced garlic
1 tbsp. chopped fresh cilantro or parsley
1 tsp. olive oil
3 plum tomatoes, diced
1 cup diced fresh pumpkin
$^1/_2$ yellow squash, diced
$^1/_2$ zucchini, diced
$^1/_2$ cup whole-kernel corn
5 cups low-sodium vegetable broth, skimmed
$^1/_2$ cup wild rice, cooked

In a large saucepan or Dutch oven over medium heat, sauté the carrot, celery, onion, garlic, and cilantro in oil and 2 tbsp. of the vegetable broth until onion is translucent. Add the remaining vegetables; sauté 3 minutes more, stirring occasionally. Add the remaining vegetable broth; bring to a boil. Reduce heat to low; simmer 30 minutes. Stir in the wild rice.

Makes 6 $1^1/_2$-cup servings. Per serving: calories 85; fat 2 g; cholesterol 0 mg; carbohydrate 15 g; protein 2.5 g.

Hot Spinach Salad

$^1/_4$ cup thinly sliced red onion
1 tbsp. chopped garlic
1 tbsp. olive oil
$^3/_4$ cup sliced mushrooms
$^1/_3$ cup balsamic vinegar
1 roasted red pepper, cut into strips
$^1/_2$ cup snow peas, sliced crosswise in thirds
1 lb. fresh spinach, trimmed and washed

In a medium skillet over high heat, sauté the onion and garlic in the oil 2 minutes. Add the mushrooms and vinegar. Reduce heat to low; simmer until the mushrooms and onions are tender. Add the roasted pepper and snow peas; cook over high heat 1 minute. Remove from heat, and toss with the spinach in a large bowl until well coated. Serve immediately on a warm plate.

Makes 2 servings. Per serving: calories 160; fat 7 g; cholesterol 0 mg; carbohydrates 18 g; protein 7 g.

> *"I believe that it's better to be looked*
> *over than it is to be overlooked."*
> —Mae West

❦ *Chapter 17* ❦
HOME SPA DAYS

For two summers in a row I spent a week in Southhampton, Long Island, at the beautiful estate of a family who turned their home into a spa for seven magical days. They invited friends and relatives from all over the country and Europe to join them for exercise, spa food, massages, spa treatments, and togetherness. I performed treatments in the pool house; Melissa taught fitness classes in the pool or out on the expansive lawn; Colin prepared the food in a restaurant-sized kitchen; and we all ate together at a table set for twenty. By the end of the week, the guests were revitalized, relaxed, and deeply grateful to the hosts, who had spared no expense in providing an incredible home spa experience.

An entire week of at-home spa pleasures is probably an unrealistic goal for most of us. But how about just a day? You want to look the best you can look, to be the healthiest you can be, and there's no better way to achieve that goal than to treat yourself to eight straight hours of spa services, spa food, and spa activities. A full day at some of the upscale destination spas mentioned in this book or even at some day spas in your neighborhood can cost hun-

The Royal Treatment

207

dreds of dollars. The equally luxurious experience you can create for yourself at home will cost only a fraction of that.

Chances are that you'll find a few spare hours here and there to try out the fabulous indulgences described in the preceding pages, to treat yourself to the world of Conscious Pleasures that is always just a moment away. But on special occasions like birthdays or anniversaries or during a stay-at-home vacation, you'll find yourself with an entire special day that you'd like to dedicate to You, or to Someone Special. In that lucky circumstance, you're going to need a plan.

By now, you have everything you need to create wonderful spa treatments for yourself and your family at home. All the tools have been provided:

1. Step-by-step explanations of more than thirty key spa treatments
2. Inspiration from top experts at the best spas
3. Basic inexpensive supplies like wool blankets and insulators
4. A few high-quality products like oils, lotions, salts, and powders
5. Spa recipes for breakfast, lunch, and dinner

All you have to do now is put the ingredients together. This may sound like an intimidating task at first, but it is actually quite simple. In order to make your Spa Day as easy to organize as possible, we're going to limit the wealth of choices by creating three different Spa Days, each with its own list of treatments:

- The Beauty/Pampering Day
- The Fitness Day
- The Detox Day

Some Suggestions for All of Your Spa Days

- Prepare some of your food the day before, so you're not rushed during your Spa Day. Some simple slicing and dicing will put you ahead of schedule. Complete recipes for breakfast, lunch, and dinner for each day are found in Chapter 16.

- Include a minimum of thirty minutes of mild aerobic exercise, such as walking or swimming, no matter which type of Spa Day you've chosen.

- Let the answering machine pick up your phone calls.

- Tell your friends you'll be busy and cannot be disturbed.

- Either indulge yourself on your own, or share your day with someone special or with a small group. Do you have daughters? Invite them to share in your Spa Day. How about your mother? Or ask two close friends to be with you. This is bonding at its best.

- You can include the Right Books in the Spa Days by having on hand one of those volumes you've been wanting to read forever but somehow haven't been able to find the time for.

- Color Therapy can be a part of every Spa Day too. Add mood and specialness to your experience with dramatic or soothing splashes of color.

- If weather permits, spend part of your Spa Day outdoors. Perhaps a lunch taken outside, or a walk, or just a few minutes admiring the sky.

- And don't forget the simplest thing—have your cushy, comfortable robe close by. Fuzzy slippers are nice too.

No exact time guidelines are given in the following descriptions because a Spa Day should be relaxing and fun. But whenever possible, do the treatments in the order they are mentioned. Certain treatments bring more benefits when experienced in proper order. For example, a massage should come after an Herbal Wrap because massage oil applied before a wrap would make detoxification through the pores more difficult.

Day One: The Beauty/Pampering Day

You'll want to use this Spa Day to look the absolute best you can, to turn yourself into a queen. Afterward, be prepared for the effects of an entire day focused on luxury and beauty. . . . Don't be surprised when others notice your glow, when they look you over with an appreciative, curious eye, wondering, "How come *she* looks so relaxed and alive?"

As you've been learning, you *deserve* this level of pleasure. Now is the time to prove it to yourself. The treatments for this Spa Day are put together to re-create that certain "flowing" sensation that spa guests report after days filled with healthy indulgences. When it's over, your skin will be polished smooth, your face glowing, and your every fiber surrendered to pleasure.

Be sure to get a good night's rest. Then, feeling refreshed, you can start this day as they do at most of the big destination spas, with an invigorating walk, a swim, or a bike ride that lasts half an hour. (Move indoors for your exercise in case of inclement weather.) This should be done at a light pace, just enough to get your heart rate into the aerobic zone. A little exercise before breakfast gets the metabolism working for the rest of the day. Then enjoy your breakfast of Banana Bran Muffins and an orange, rich in vitamin C, which is good for the skin. After a brief rest get into the mood by preparing the Body Scrub that you learned in Chapter 3. Make sure to have all the ingredients close at hand so you'll stay warm. (Dashing out of the room to fetch a loofah can be a chilling experience.) You can take a break afterward or, if you like, segue directly into a Love Wrap. (If you choose to perform these treatments back to back, omit the final application of cream in the Body Scrub. Transfer yourself or your partner onto your spa sheet, and proceed with the anointing and wrapping procedure you learned in Chapter 9.) A Love Wrap feels especially warm and loving when it's preceded by the slightly cooling Body Scrub. Of course, your attitude and intention and love count more than any technique. Just be there, and care, and that will be enough. You'll see.

By now it will be mid- to late morning, a perfect time to sit and enjoy your partner or the companionship of the Right Book that you've stowed away for this occasion.

When lunchtime approaches and you set the table and spread out the healthy spa dishes—Butternut Squash Soup and Grilled Chicken Caesar Salad—focus on Conscious Pleasure Principle Number 1—Preparation. The buildup to the pleasure of eating is often as great as the meal itself. The combination of spa treatments and exercise leaves almost everyone ravenous, but don't rush it. Take your time. Enjoy!

After lunch, take some time to digest, and then start back in with the facial from Chapter 6. Even though it's called the Gentleman's Facial, that doesn't mean it necessarily has to be for a man. But if you women can get husbands or boyfriends to join you for a Spa Day, you're in for a unique day of togetherness. Afterward, no matter who receives the facial, make sure to glance in the mirror for a little Conscious Pleasure Principle Number 7—Gratitude. Be grateful to yourself for taking the time to care about beauty. Rest in your robe, just enjoying the scenery for a little while.

For your seaweed (Chapter 11) and hydrotherapy (Chapter 4) experiences later in the afternoon, you'll head to your own private spa wet room, otherwise known as the bathroom, for a wrap and a soak that will leave you limp. You can apply the Seaweed Self-Wrap directly in the tub and then be ready for the bath that follows. Take time to rest then, stretching out with your book.

Your dinner of Smoked Turkey Quesadilla, Spa Avocado Salsa, and Black Bean Relish is filled with unprocessed goodness that will keep you glowing on the inside as well as the outside.

For snacks on this day, have a cantaloupe at midmorning and an Apple-Pear Salad in the afternoon.

Step by Step

- a half hour of light aerobic exercise
- breakfast
- Body Scrub (Chapter 3)
- Love Wrap (Chapter 9)
- lunch
- facial (Chapter 6)
- Seaweed Self-Wrap (Chapter 11)
- Hydrotherapy Bath (chapter 4)
- dinner

Day Two:
The Fitness Day

This can be a physically challenging day for you!

After an hour of aerobic movement (walking, jogging, cycling, swimming, rowing, aerobics class, etc.) first thing in the morning to get the muscles thoroughly warmed up and the metabolism going, have a breakfast of Bran Crepes with Fruited Cottage Cheese Filling, which is high in carbohydrates and B vitamins—essential for high-energy exercising. At midmorning offer your feet a little relief with a Foot Treatment like the one described in Chapter 12. This will help soothe soles made sore by the extra pounding of exercise.

Your hair usually takes a beating of its own when you exercise, whether it is caused by wind, sunlight, or excess washing. With the Hot Oil Hair Pack from Chapter 12 you'll replenish shine and body while giving yourself a break from your demanding schedule today.

When your tummy tells you to start thinking about lunch, you can look forward to enjoying the Guava Barbecued Shrimp and Wildberry Cheesecake, with its wholesome goodness and satisfying stock of carbohydrates. But first go for another half hour of exercise, concentrating on your abdominal muscles and buns this time, doing sit-ups and leg lifts and crunches and knee raises until you can "feel the burn."

After lunch, rest. Feel for the muscles that are the most tight or sore from all the activity, and focus on them with a Sport Fango. Actually, applying any heated clay, mud, or even seaweed is going to do wonders for your aching limbs. When this is rinsed off, you can head for the gym! If you have some weights at your home spa, by all means stay there and use them, but if you don't, this is a perfect opportunity to explore a membership at the local club if you don't already have one. The fitness experts there can guide you through the kind of muscle-mass-building exercises that are mentioned in the last part of this chapter.

Then do what everyone does after achieving exhaustion at the big spas: book your massage appointment for late in the afternoon. That way you can end your day of physical exertion with some major physical pleasure and slide off the massage table directly toward the dinner table. Your final meal of Spa Rolls, Fusilli Marco Polo, and skim milk contains all the elements needed to replenish your body after so much exertion.

Step by Step

- an hour of aerobic exercise
- breakfast
- Foot Treatment (Chapter 12)
- Hot Oil Hair Pack (Chapter 12)
- calisthenics
- lunch
- Sport Fango (Chapter 15)
- an hour of weight training (Chapter 17)
- full-body Spa Massage (Chapter 8)
- dinner

Day Three:
The Detox Day

Don't be fooled by the treatments on this day; even though they're every bit as pleasurable as the other days, their detoxifying effects are also quite powerful. For that reason, it is extra important that you *drink at least two quarts of pure water* during this day. The reason for this is that, as a result of these treatments, your body may begin the process of purging itself of waste products. The water helps flush them through the system—from your cells to your bloodstream to your liver and kidneys, and then to elimination. This detoxifying is especially pronounced in your lymph glands and vessels, which benefit greatly from the extra water intake.

This will be the most "spiritual" of your Spa Days because you are distancing yourself from the everyday world of overconsumption. When you purge your body, you lighten your spirit as well, without fail. Therefore start this day with a Meditation experience like the one described in Chapter 10. Center yourself on your desire for health and purity for the first half hour of the morning, before you've done anything but wash your face and hands in the bathroom. After this, engage in any kind of exercise that is going to warm you up. Do some yoga or other stretches that open the joints and improve circulation. Wear extra sweatpants and sweatshirts. The idea is to get yourself sweating and purging before any of the treatments even begin. If you exercise indoors, turn the heat up or the air conditioner down.

Your breakfast consists of a Tropical Smoothie, which will be enough to fuel your body for several hours without adding anything heavy to work off. If you get hungry during the day, have a snack of fresh carrot sticks, apple slices, or rice cakes. After resting a little, begin preparations for the Herbal Wrap. If you have a steam room or sauna or Jacuzzi available, by all means use it to raise your core body temperature. A hot shower will do fine too. Once again the key here is heat. Apply the Herbal Wrap for twenty to thirty minutes, making sure you or your partner has water to drink through a straw and that a cold compress is applied when wanted to the forehead and face. If you are doing this Spa Day on your own, try the Tummy Wrap, also explained in Chapter 5.

Make sure to take plenty of time to rest after the Herbal Wrap, which is one of the most intense spa treatments. Recline for twenty minutes afterward, preferably out in the fresh air, without washing the herbs off.

Next, after you've given yourself plenty of time to recover, prepare for the Journey (either the Self or the Partner version), from Chapter 10. Treatments of this nature are part of the Ayurvedic cleansing program known as *panchakarma,* which is practiced at Dr. Chopra's Center for Well Being. Since you've already prepared the skin by an application of herbs, you do not have to be too aggressive with the loofah-scrubbing part of this treatment. But make sure not to skimp when it comes to the *Shirodhara* head massage—it's incredible.

Lunch is Chilled Fruit Soup and a Garden Pocket Melt, another light meal chosen to help the body as it naturally sheds impurities. After sufficient rest, start your afternoon with a Foot Treatment (reflexology) from Chapter 12. This can be a self-reflexology if you're enjoying a Spa Day alone. When you're finished, apply the Herbal Inhalation from Chapter 5. This deep cleansing of the respiratory system also benefits the nerves and skin.

Now, more exercise. This is the toughest Spa Day, meant to purge your system and clean you out. So it's back into the sweats for another half hour of heat-inducing movement, whichever kind you've chosen. Then, as a reward for all your hard work this day, sit back and enjoy a long hot Clay Foot Soak from Chapter 15. Not only will it ease your tired feet, but the clay will also draw out impurities through the pores on your soles.

Dinner is Vegetable Harvest Soup and Hot Spinach Salad, a perfect light combination to nourish your body while keeping it pumping out impurities till bedtime.

Step by Step

- Meditation (Chapter 10)
- stretching and warmth-inducing exercise
- breakfast
- Herbal Wrap (Chapter 5)
- Home Journey (Chapter 10)
- lunch
- reflexology (Chapter 12)
- Herbal Inhalation (Chapter 5)
- more warming exercise
- Clay Foot Soak (Chapter 15)
- dinner

Home Gym Setup

If nothing else, the physical exhaustion you feel after a sweaty go at the StairMaster or forty-five minutes spent with Jane Fonda makes the experience of spa treatments even more luxurious than they are normally. Imagine immersing yourself in a hot Seaweed Bath and feeling the ache of well-used muscles dissolve in blissful mineralized warmth. This is reason enough to make at least a small investment in some home fitness equipment.

If you have the space available in your home (perhaps a child's bedroom after they've moved out on their own?), stocking it with a few choice pieces of exercise equipment may be just the incentive you need to keep yourself toned and fit throughout the year. On the other hand, you can squeeze a stationary bike into just about any corner; a separate room for the purpose is definitely not necessary.

Mike Angus, spa director at the Polo Club in Boca Raton, Florida, says that the most important thing for anyone to remember when they are planning an exercise area in their own home is that it be a comfortable, attractive space for them to spend time in.

His clientele are among the most health conscious in the country. Boca Raton is known for 365 days a year of sporting activities, and Polo Club guests expect the best, whether they're working out at the state-of-the-art facility or following their own fitness regimen at home.

Mike is a tall, angular Canadian who practices what he preaches, keeping his six-foot frame lean and healthy through a regular regimen of cross-training. "Nobody would work out at all if they didn't like their environment or their training partner," he asserts in his unhurried Canadian accent. "In fact, the one thing I've seen more of recently is the phenomenon of the personal trainer. The fact is that people just don't like working so hard at something like weight training. With the trainer there it's psychologically not as difficult, almost as if somebody else were doing the workout for them, which they would actually prefer if it were possible." Mike smiles, and a good-natured but shrewd understanding of his customers is evident.

According to Mike, weight training is definitely the wave of the future in the fitness world. "There has been an amazing change recently," he states. "Our revenues from the personal training department have almost quadrupled in the past two years, and it's all due to people wanting to put on more muscle mass, which has been proven to increase their metabolism and functional strength. In the old days all people wanted was cardio, and now it's more of a combination. We recommend thirty minutes of cardio, twenty of weight training, and ten of stretching for the average person's workout. The weight lifting has been shown to make people stronger, even when they're in their eighties."

When shopping for your home gym, look for fitness specialty stores in the Yellow Pages, usually under "Exercise Equipment—Sales and Service." Many home gym options are available, with up-front investments ranging from fifty dollars for a set of basic dumbbells and a floor mat to over fifty thousand for track lighting, a sound system, aerobic floors, cardio equipment, biodynamic multistation gyms, free weights, benches, stretching equipment, and more.

Remember one thing: When it comes to fitness, the most important ingredient for success is enthusiasm. A well-lit room full of the latest equipment is not going to get you into better shape—*you* are. The most precious currency in the fitness world is time and the willingness to do what it takes.

You are going to find, if you take the time to treat yourself royally with the spa services in this book—spending an hour on massage every other week, cleansing your pores with exfoliation, or soaking up the effects of nurturing herbs—that you will naturally have more energy and inclination to exercise as well. When the urge hits, don't deny it. A brisk half-hour walk through the neighborhood is all it takes to gain an edge on fitness. But if it's cold outside, and you've decided to put together some exercise equipment for your own home gym, the following resources may help you.

Cardio Equipment

Life Fitness	(800) 735-3867
StairMaster	(800) 782-4799
Trotter	(800) 677-6544
NordicTrack	(800) 892-2174

Weight Machines

Cybex	(516) 585-9000
Koist	(800) 548-5438
Ivanko	(800) 247-9044
Vectra Fitness	(800) 283-2872

Exercise Mats

Bollinger	(800) 527-1166

Conclusion

As you go about creating your own home spa environment, remember the lessons that you've been taught by the healers, spa therapists, doctors, spa directors, and spa owners in this book. Each one of them has added a little gem about health or beauty or luxury to help you on the way to creating a healthy, pleasure-filled lifestyle.

Spa Lessons

1. Veronica at Sans Souci taught us we've "got to keep the folks warm."

2. Wesley at Ihilani in Hawaii taught us about the importance of Mother Earth and Mother Ocean, that we're all connected on this planet of waters.

3. At the Golden Door we learned the power of working with fresh natural herbs.

4. Maggie at the Phoenician pointed out how important it is to treat your man royally once in a while with a facial.

5. A special guest at the Doral Spa showed us how to receive therapeutic touch in a full-body Spa Massage.

6. Susan at Enchantment explained the most important technique of all, the "Love Technique."

7. Dr. Deepak Chopra at the Chopra Center for Well Being taught us that "people come to spas for one thing—improving the quality of their life."

8. Tonya at Canyon Ranch showed us that spa services can be one of the highest forms of giving and that seaweed has some surprisingly powerful properties.

9. At the Green Valley Spa we learned to use color to add brightness to our days and to read the Right Books to uplift our spirits. Plus we learned to take care of the whole, from top to toe, with Kim's hair treatment and Marianne's foot treatment.

10. Jeanie at Meadowood demonstrated a modern-day version of a classic French aristocratic experience using Chardonnay grape extracts and aromatherapy.

11. Larry at the Camelback taught us to "slow down enough to enjoy the treatment."

12. Cheryl at the PGA Resort and Spa taught us how simple it can be to prepare delicious and guilt-free dishes in our own kitchens—how we can "take out the fat, not the flavor."

13. Mike Angus shared some wisdom about the prevailing trends in spa health and fitness, offering advice for those seeking to continue exercising at home.

And don't forget the Conscious Pleasure Principles! They'll come in handy again and again, not just in your experiences with spas but in every aspect of your life.

1. **Preparation:** Plan time for yourself. You're worth it.

2. **Ambience:** Notice and soak in the beauty in your life.

3. **Greetings:** Honor and appreciate the people you meet.

4. **Letting Go:** Consciously release tension, worry, and stress.

5. **Immersion:** Concentrate on the moment. It's all you've got.

6. **Surrendering to Pleasure:** Be good to yourself. Don't fight it.

7. **Gratitude:** Allow life to fill you up. It will overflow to others.

Enjoying conscious pleasure in your life is the main message I hope you've heard while reading this book. Spas can teach you many things about yourself, about your needs, your vulnerabilities, and your strengths. You need to be taken care of periodically, and you also need to take care of others. You inhabit a fragile body that must be treated well. When you begin to truly treasure your health and your vitality, you will automatically seek out those places that can fulfill your desire for conscious pleasure.

Spas offer such an opportunity. They are sanctuaries that support you in your quest for love and health. To not take advantage of their growing popularity and accessibility would be to waste a precious resource. To not create your own spa sanctum at home once in a while would be to overlook a priceless gift that lies right before you all the time. It would be to overlook your Self.

Love yourself. Give yourself the royal treatment.

Appendix A
SPA TOOLS

You may want to purchase a few additional items to comple-
ment the basic necessities of a home spa program. Everything
you absolutely need was listed in Chapter 2. The following ancil-
lary products and tools will add to your enjoyment when and if you
decide to acquire them. For information about these and many
other home spa products, call Tara Spa Therapies at (888) 868-
2433. You can also contact the International Spa and Fitness Association (ISPA) directly at (703) 838-2930 to discover a wide range
of other manufacturers and suppliers of spa products and equipment. Make sure to contact them if you plan on opening a spa
yourself.

The Royal Treatment Home Spa "Conscious Pleasure Kit"

Everything you'll need to perform the treatments described in this
book is contained in one package. Three options are available,
ranging from a beginner's set of basic products to a complete offering that includes everything you'll need to immerse yourself in
an all-inclusive home spa experience.

Optional
Equipment

Paraffin Bath: About the size of a large shoebox, this unit warms up blocks of paraffin wax to the perfect temperature for immersing hands or feet. Some advanced spa treatments include "painting" the hot wax over a person's whole body and wrapping them in gauze. The warm wax sends penetrating heat into the muscles and joints while at the same time leaving the skin soft and supple.

Massage Table: If you have the space and it fits your budget, a professional, portable massage table is an excellent item to have in a home spa. It folds up like a large suitcase, and when opened, it provides a comfortable cushioned surface on which to lie during massages and spa treatments. It makes treatments easier on the person *giving* them as well, since the adjustable height of the table makes it no longer necessary to bend over or kneel above the partner.

Hot Towel Cabi: In order to keep your towels steamy hot for use in the home spa treatments, you'll need to keep them well insulated. One upscale alternative to your Spa Thermal Unit is the Hot Towel Cabi from Italy, a sleek enameled unit that keeps a dozen moist towels hot indefinitely.

Hydrocollator: A heavy-duty stainless steel heating unit, this piece of equipment is used in many spas to warm towels and herbal sheets. It is also ideal for keeping clays, seaweeds, and other products warm.

Steam Unit: Various steam units appropriate for the home are available today. One type fits over the top of a massage table like a tent. Another uses aromatherapy oil inside a plastic steam capsule big enough to fit one person. And Russian steam baths, the type where the person's head is exposed at the top, are still popular.

Aromatherapy Pillows: The same heat-retaining pillow placed over guests' necks and shoulders at the Chopra Center for Well Being can be purchased for use at home. Also, a line of Eye Pillows and Hand Mitts is available, filled with a blend of gently aromatic herbs to soothe the senses.

Seaweeds: Most seaweed compounds that you'll find at cosmetics counters contain several other ingredients as well. For the purest form of the product, it's best to purchase it in its freeze-dried powdered form and then reconstitute it yourself.

Bulk Herbs: Picking your own herbs and combining them yourself is ideal, but most of us won't be able to find the time for that. Several companies provide preblended mixtures for specific purposes. Two were mentioned at the end of Chapter 5.

Muds and Clays: The mud found in your backyard after a rainstorm just won't do for therapeutic purposes. Some of the muds sold in beauty supply stores may contain additives. A pure unadulterated source is what's used in spas.

Moisturizing Lotions: Hundreds of products are available, but most of them contain a lot of unnatural ingredients. A few manufacturers specialize in creating lotions from pure sources, perfect for spa applications. I recommend Alba brand lotions in particular; they can be found in many spas.

Appendix B
MORE GREAT SPAS

Many of my favorite spas were not even mentioned in *The Royal Treatment* due to a lack of space. Others were not included because they are hot springs resorts rather than true spas. The range of healthy retreats available to you grows every month of the year, and I want to include at least a partial list of some of them here. They are all definitely worth visiting if you ever have the opportunity.

The list is by no means complete. For an extensive overview of all the major spa resorts in America and several abroad, consult Bernard Burt's *Healthy Escapes,* published each year by Fodor's. And if you're thinking about a spa vacation, make sure to call one of the travel agencies that specialize in spa packages. The best two such agencies in business are Spa Finders at (212) 924-6800 and Spa Trek Travel at (212) 779-3480.

Watercourse Way, Palo Alto, California (415) 462-2000
An urban retreat based on the theme of water.

Harbin Hot Springs, Middletown, California (707) 987-2477
A clothing-optional environment with natural hot springs, a blissful warm pool, cold streams, great massages, and plenty of nature all

around. The atmosphere is so peaceful here that wild deer walk among the people.

Orr Hot Springs, Ukiah, California (707) 462-6277
A remote, secluded sanctuary nestled in the redwoods with natural waters, communal kitchen, sauna, and private tubs, on a quiet forest lane.

The Greenhouse, Dallas, Texas, and Palm Beach, Florida (817) 640-4000
One of the truly luxurious luxury spas, built by Neiman Marcus and Charles of the Ritz. An all-women retreat, this is first class all the way.

Hilton Waikoloa, Hawaii (808) 885-1234
A great resort on the Big Island, famous among honeymooners and spa goers alike. You can swim with the dolphins and explore new high-tech spa treatments.

Grand Wailea, Maui (808) 875-1234
One of the most gorgeous properties in the world. They've fashioned a dream spa filled with magic waters and fantastic treatments in one of the most beautiful settings imaginable.

Ten Thousand Waves, Santa Fe, New Mexico (505) 988-1047
A day spa on the outskirts of Santa Fe, this retreat features views of some breathtaking scenery right from your hot tub. Excellent massage staff, private pools, kimonos worn by the guests.

Gurney's Inn, Montauk, New York (516) 668-2345
A traditional spa haven on the tip of Long Island—one of the very few to employ real seawater in their treatments.

The Spa at the Peaks, Telluride, Colorado (970) 728-6800
Gorgeous setting and fabulous spa. Ideal for a ski/spa getaway package.

Norwich Inn, Norwich, Connecticut (203) 886-2401
Homey and luxurious, a 1920s country inn turned spa, only two hours north of New York City.

Cal-a-Vie, Vista, California (619) 945-2055
Exclusive and serious about their health regimen, this southern California spa is limited to twenty-four guests a week.

Miraval, Tucson, Arizona (520) 825-4000
A spa with a mission—to turn your life around with mind-expanding experiences, plus the usual luxury and service.

And just in case you become inspired to visit one of the spas featured in this book, here's a quick list of contact numbers:

Sans Souci, Ocho Rios, Jamaica (800) 203-7456

Ihilani, Oahu, Hawaii (800) 626-4446

The Sonoma Mission Inn, Sonoma, California (800) 862-4945

The Golden Door, Escondido, California (619) 744-5777

The Phoenician, Scottsdale, Arizona (800) 888-8234

The Doral Spa, Miami, Florida (800) 331-7768

Enchantment Resort, Sedona, Arizona (800) 826-4180

Chopra Center for Well Being, La Jolla, California (888) 424-6772

Canyon Ranch—Berkshires, Lenox, Massachusetts (800) 742-9000

Green Valley Spa, Saint George, Utah (800) 237-1068

Meadowood Resort and Spa, Saint Helena, California (800) 458-8080

Camelback Inn, Phoenix, Arizona (800) 242-2635

PGA Resort and Spa, West Palm Beach, Florida (800) THE-SPA5

The Polo Club, Boca Raton, Florida (561) 995-1250

Index

Olive oil, 148
Omaha Indians, 19
Orange, 169
O'Rourke, Maureen, 45
Orr Hot Springs, Ukiah, California, 228
Our Earth, Our Cure (Dextreit), 186

P

Panchakarma, 121, 215
Papaya Facial Blend, 62, 66, 67
    recipe for, 64
Paraffin bath, 150, 155, 224
Partner's Foot Treatment, 105
Pear, Apple, Raisin Compote, 196
Peliotherapy, 178
Peloids, 178
Peppermint, 51, 147, 148, 168–169, 184
Percussion, 79, 81, 86, 87, 89, 95
PGA Resort and Spa, West Palm Beach, Florida, 187–189, 220, 230
Phoenician, Scottsdale, Arizona, 60–63, 219, 229
Pine, 169
Pineal gland, 124
Pineapple, 62
Pineapple Teriyaki Sauce, 198
Pinpoint pressure, 77, 79, 85–87, 90, 91, 93–95
Pliny, 178
Polo Club, Boca Raton, Florida, 216, 217, 230
Potassium chloride, 22
Powdered clay, 36
Prakruti, 121
Preparation, 8, 211, 220
Prophet, The, 157
Pueblo People Wrap, 110
Pule, 32
Puyallup-Nisqually Indians, 19

R

Recipes, 209
    Apple-Pear Salad, 194
    Avocado Salsa, 194
    Banana Bran Muffins, 191
    Banana Salsa, 198–199
    Black Bean Relish, 193–194
    Bran Crepes with Fruited Cottage Cheese Filling, 195–196
    Butternut Squash Soup, 191–192
    Caesar Dressing, 192–193
    Chilled Fruit Soup, 203
    Energy Bar, 201–202
    exfoliant, 22–23
    Fruit Puree, 197
    Fusilli Marco Polo, 200–201
    Garden Pocket Melt, 204
    Grilled Chicken Caesar Salad, 192
    Guava Barbecue Sauce, 198
    Guava Barbecued Shrimp, 197
    Hot Spinach Salad, 205–206
    Papaya Facial Blend, 64
    Pear, Apple, Raisin Compote, 196
    Pineapple Teriyaki Sauce, 198
    Smoked Turkey Quesadilla, 193
    Soy Sauce, 204
    Spa Rolls, 200
    Tropical Smoothie, 203
    Vegetable Harvest Soup, 205
    Wildberry Cheesecake, 199
Redfield, James, 157
Reflexology, 150–157, 215
Remineralization, 136
Return of the Rishi (Chopra), 131
Robes, 13, 69–72
Rolls, 200, 213
Romans, 18, 38
Rose, 169
Rose, Jeanne, 175
Rosehip, 110, 113
Rosemary, 49, 51, 169